"Dr. Kuttner's excellent new book provides logical and scientific explanations on how the body and the mind together create chronic pain, and it offers practical and effective solutions on how to decrease and release it. Dr. Kuttner's book, which is based on decades of his clinical experience, is a true gift of hope and promise to the countless people, who have been feeling trapped in their own bodies."

Dr. Friedemann Schaub, author of the USA Best-Book Award Winner 'Fear and Anxiety Solution'.

"In his new book, Dr. Kuttner does a wonderful job explaining acute and chronic pain. As he emphasizes, understanding is the first step to relieving pain. His book is full of clear, easy-to-understand explanations and diagrams. You, Pain Free has a toolbox full of practical tips and techniques pain sufferers can use. This book is a must read for people with chronic pain who have not found relief with conventional methods."

- David Schechter, M.D. Pain Medicine/Sports Medicine specialist, Beverly Hills, California, USA Author, *Think Away Your Pain: Your brain is the solution to your pain*

First Printing, 2017

ISBN: 9781520363486

Life After Pain Ltd

12 Beach Road
Papakura, 2113
New Zealand

www.LifeAfterPain.com

This book is not intended as a substitute for the medical advice of physicians. The reader should regularly consult a physician in matters relating to his/her health and particularly with respect to any symptoms that may require diagnosis or medical attention. Names and identifying details have been changed to protect the privacy of individuals.

Bonus Material on www.6KeysPainFree.com

-

Life After Pain

6 Keys to Break Free of Chronic
Pain and Get Your Life Back

For Eira,
who rocks.

Contents

FOREWORD

If you want to end your chronic pain once and for all, this book is for you.

In this book, you'll learn three things. You'll discover why everything you've tried so far hasn't worked. You'll learn a totally different approach that does work. And finally, you will receive the six keys you need to dismantle each part of the chronic pain cycle.

This practical knowledge is what I used to end seven years of back pain, and since then it's helped thousands of other people get their lives back from chronic pain.

It's now your turn to get out of pain and get back to being the happy, active person you used to be. What you're going to learn is simple, but not always easy. However, for the people that consistently apply this in their life – it works.

1

The Journey Begins

I stood poised on the edge of a three-hundred-foot cliff overlooking the wild ocean of New Zealand. The wind buffeted me as I readied to launch my hang glider. My son, Benjamin, was there helping me.

"The wind's a little northerly," Benjamin said. "And it's getting up a bit. Are you sure about this?"

"It'll be fine," I said.

I pushed forward on the hang glider bar and leapt into space, feeling a drop in the pit of my stomach as the wind lifted me high into the air. It was exhilarating – blue skies, wind rushing in my face… I was in my paradise.

But as I struggled to level the wings, I realised I was already twenty meters behind my take-off point and rapidly going up and backwards. The wind was too strong and I was being driven up a deep cut between the hills and away from the safe zone.

I was faced with two choices: I could pull in the bar and slowly fight my way down into the wind, then work my way around the front of the hills to gain height. This was the slower and safer option.

Or, I could push the bar forward and allow myself to continue upwards and backwards away from the sea. This short cut would take me over an outcrop of the cliffs. I would be quite low and close to the hills but I thought this was an acceptable risk.

In that moment, I made a decision that would change the course of my life. I chose the short cut.

I pushed the bar forward and felt the earth drop away again as the glider sped upwards. As I came over the brow of the hill alarm bells began to ring frantically in my head. I saw the ground below me fell into a small hidden valley. This was a dangerous situation. The valley below could easily cause an air rotor that would plunge me downwards.

And then the wind, which had previously lifted me, hit my left wing like a breaking wave. From a height of fifty feet I plummeted towards the ground at top speed.

Instinctively I pushed the bar out and turned the dive into a swoop. A foot lower, I would probably have died. A foot higher, I would have had the ride of my life. Instead, I hit the ground almost perfectly parallel, ploughing into the earth at maximum velocity. The aluminium bars of my glider shattered around me and I felt the huge impact rip through my body as my world exploded in *pain*.

The glider flipped over and I found myself lying on my back with the glider on top of me. I couldn't breathe and felt strangely floaty. And it was there, lying still in total darkness, unable to move or breathe, that I had the clearest thought: *I'm about to die.* In that moment, I wasn't upset by this. It was simply the way things were.

Floating in the void, I then heard a disembodied voice above me.

"Excuse me, sir. Can I lift this off you and turn you into the recovery position?"

The twisted hang glider was lifted, and I opened my eyes. Above me stood not an angel but an off-road trail biker. He started to roll me on my side and the pain exploded again. My shoulders and collar bones were no longer attached to my body. All the joints had been dislocated.

I hugged myself, hanging onto whatever I could, and he gently helped me to sit. My son Benjamin's concerned face suddenly appeared.

"Are you ok?" he said. Then he and the angelic trail biker (I never found out his name) helped me stand, and with waves of agony rolling over me, I climbed down the hill.

It was the longest walk of my life. Each step was pure pain. At the bottom of the hill I had to climb up through another gully to get to the road. I still remember the relative bliss as I leant against the reclined seat in my car and Benjamin drove me to the doctor, trying to miss the many bumps on the old road from the beach.

* * *

With my shoulders and ribs heavily strapped, I left the emergency room and hobbled home. I spent a total of one week off work. At the time I had a busy medical practice out in the country. I was a family doctor and presided over everything from births, deaths, minor operations, car crashes and the proverbial sick child in the middle of the night.

It was a blessing in disguise that taking more time off to recover never even occurred to me. I limped into work on a Monday morning, drugged up on painkillers, with my dislocated shoulder strapped up, and a herniated disc forming a hot ball of pain at the base of my spine that sent shooting pains down my leg.

I let it all wash over me – the pain, the busy demands of work, the drugged up semi-conscious nights. I dug deep, struggled, and somehow managed to hold it all together until the weekend. And then I did it all over again the next week. And the next. And the next.

After many months the pain in my shoulders and collarbone settled and I was able to move around more easily. But it slowly dawned on me that the pain in my lower back was not getting better. It was still there – strong as ever – many months after my medical training told me it should be easing.

This is a stage anyone who's had chronic pain will know. It is the slow and wrenching realisation that things are not as they should be.

Each day was a struggle. I found myself slipping into an existence I could only describe as 'grey'. I would grit my teeth and make it to the weekend. If I did something I loved, like gardening or playing tennis, my enjoyment was dulled by the sure knowledge I would pay for it later with days of intense pain.

The injuries from my crash sent me on a journey of more than seven years – deep into the valley of darkness that is chronic pain. However, I have journeyed out the other side of that place, and I can tell you there is light at the end of it. Since the day I fell out of the sky I've not only been able to heal my own chronic pain, I've helped many, many others do the same.

In this book you're going to discover how to create your vehicle out of pain.

The keys to getting back your life from chronic pain are both simple and profound. Bear in mind though, simple may not mean easy. The first step is understanding what is *really* happening when your pain 'should' have improved but hasn't.

To begin, I invite you to step on the path with me and let us move onward together.

People usually make a few false starts before they step confidently on the true journey out of pain.

Perhaps, like I did, you started to shop around once you realised your pain was not improving. This is when the hunt for the diagnosis begins. If you have an awful pain **that's not going away, there must be a reason for it. And** you're going to find it so you can fix it.

At this stage you may see your primary healthcare practitioner and be discouraged when the only help you receive is a prescription for stronger painkillers. You may go to other specialists – orthopaedic surgeons, chiropractors, osteopaths, acupuncturists – always searching...

This is perfectly natural. The only thing worse than having awful pain that's not going away, is having that pain and not knowing the reason for it. This leaves you open to anxiety – you imagine the worst – and hopelessness, because it seems you're suffering for no reason.

Victor Frankl was a Jewish psychiatrist interred in a Nazi concentration camp during World War II. He observed that people who could not find meaning in their suffering soon died. He said:

"If there is meaning in life at all, then there must be meaning in suffering."

If you cannot find a cause for your pain then you lose the meaning for your suffering and it becomes harder to bear. This is a profound driver behind the search for the diagnosis. Once you have your diagnosis, the search stops and you can get on with your life, such as it is.

* * *

For me it took seven long years of daily pain before I had the insight that set me on the road to recovery. However I know many people who have spent much longer in the half-life of chronic pain.

My first glimpse of freedom started with a small and seemingly insignificant realisation. I noticed something about how my pain behaved. Instead of thinking, *oh, it's because of this reason* and justifying it away, I looked at this small fact and thought: *This doesn't really make sense...*

What I noticed was that I had terrible pain every morning, significant pain in the evening, pain at night and pain on the weekends. But I had hardly any pain when I was busy at work.

Up to this point I accepted the diagnosis for my pain. It made perfect sense. I had a prolapsed disc at L5/S1, which I could see was damaged via an MRI. This was obviously the cause of my lower-back pain and sciatica.

However, my work day was full of stress, plus lots of bending, twisting and lifting – all the movements that were agony if I did them at home. Doing these movements at work mechanically stressed my damaged disc exactly the same way as they did at home.

So... if my diagnosis was correct, how was it possible I had almost no pain while at work? I thought on this long and hard and the only explanation I could find was this: *My pain was not coming from my 'damaged' disc.*

There really wasn't any other logical explanation. This was the moment I had to let go of my original diagnosis. It was difficult to do because now I was back at square one – facing pain and suffering for no reason. So I began a search to answer the next question: *Where was my pain* really *coming from?*

Now we come to the heart of the matter.

If my pain wasn't coming from my damaged disc, it must originate elsewhere. At this point, I was finally open to exploring a new possibility. You also need to be open to a completely new set of possibilities. If you are not, we cannot continue on this journey together.

To progress, you now need to let go of your current diagnosis. It's not easy. In fact, when I have this conversation with my pain clinic clients, I need to be very sensitive so they know I believe everything they've told me.

Please understand, I do not doubt your pain is real, or that you have tried everything to get rid of it. I'm not saying it's 'all in your head' or you're somehow making everything up. I can't see your expression as you read these words. However, I've been where you've been, and I know it's challenging to let go of the pain diagnosis. I know this, because I was in exactly same place for seven long years.

I had a wonderfully plausible reason for my back pain. I had slammed straight into a hillside while flying through the air. I had herniated a disc and disrupted joints all through my body.

The truth, however, was that once I was able to put all that aside and follow the path I'm going to lay out for you in this book, within six weeks my pain diminished dramatically. After twelve weeks it was gone.

The key question to answer is: will this work for you?

There are almost no guarantees in life. What I can guarantee is that if you continue on your current path, you will get the same results. From my experience these techniques have worked for shoulder pain, neck pain, chronic headaches, abdominal pain, leg pain, arm pain, face pain, and widespread pain.

The last question to answer is: should you try surgery to fix your chronic pain?

This is a difficult question, and a book can never replace a competent surgeon. However, statistics show[1,2,3] that many types of back, neck and shoulder surgery fail in bringing pain relief for one devastatingly simple reason: the surgeon never pinpointed the true source of the pain.

Every day in my clinic I see people who have chronic pain. For some of them, it started after an accident – perhaps a car accident or whiplash injury. For others, it was a minor thing like picking up a suitcase, or a missed a step that jarred their back. While some remember a day when they just woke up and the pain was there.

All of them want only one thing: for the pain to go away and never come back.

There was one patient I'll always remember. He explained the history of his pain – how it started, when it would flare, the different experts he'd seen to try and sort it out. I listened as I always try to, without jumping to conclusions or aiming for an early diagnosis, just taking it all in.

Then he stopped, and leaned back in his chair. "So, what do you think Doc?" he asked. "Can you fix me?"

"No," I said, without hesitation.

He stared at me. "What do you mean no?"

Clearly this was not going as expected. "I can't fix you," I said. "But *you* can fix yourself."

It's not that the experts you've been to so far have not been helpful. It's just that you're still in pain. The reason is that they have missed a fundamental truth – chronic pain is not just a case of treating the part that hurts. In my fifteen years of being a pain specialist I've found that there are 6 interlocking keys that you need to lift yourself out of chronic pain.

Once these keys are mastered, you take charge of your life. You regain what pain has stolen from you – your control, your peace of mind, your sense of purpose. And, bit by bit, you get back to doing the things that bring joy and meaning to your life.

Action Steps

1. What was your diagnosis? Are you willing to put this aside (even temporarily) in order to explore a new cause (and cure) for your pain?

2. Think about how your pain behaves. When you examine this, are there times you've noticed (like I did) that your pain did not completely make sense?

3. Alternately, are there times when you have little or no pain? When does this occur? And do these pain-free periods appear to have a logical cause – or not?

THE
FIRST
KEY

2

The Unexpected Tale of How Your Best Friend Became Your Worst Enemy

Welcome to the First Key for you to master in your journey out of chronic pain. This key will change your understanding of how and why you still feel pain, and allow you to explore new possibilities for pain relief.

Imagine how it would feel if your best friend, who had always been there for you, changed into your worst enemy. Even more troubling, he or she did this for no obvious reason.

Imagine your previous friend looked, moved and sounded exactly the same as always. *But...* his or her advice, which had always kept you safe, was now designed to completely destroy your life.

Another twist to this tale is that this entity lives inside you and therefore is always with you. You cannot escape their poisonous inner messages no matter where you go or what you do. In fact their advice is often loudest when you try to do the things that give you joy.

And the final kicker? You don't know this change has happened so you continue to believe the messages are true. You're suffering and you don't understand why.

In this story your best friend was your pain system. Ever since you were a little baby your pain system has kept you safe, warning you the instant your body was in danger. It has been your constant companion through all the years and while we perceive pain as an unpleasant sensation, the truth is that without it, none of us would live very long.

However, for people in chronic pain, something unexpected happens. Your pain system, which has been your most faithful ally, goes rogue and starts distorting and amplifying the messages it sends to your brain. And just like that, your best friend becomes your worst enemy.

This is one of the true giant causes of chronic pain. It is the invisible elephant in the room, and it is only in the last decade or so that scientists have been able to point to it as a primary cause of chronic pain.[1,2,3,4,5,6,7,8,9,10,11,12,13,14]

The idea that the pain you feel *may not be* related to physical damage is a difficult one. Since your birth, pain has always meant one thing – your body has been damaged and you are in danger. But if your pain system is malfunctioning, you can feel very real and sometimes excruciating pain, with no physical damage being present.

The most extreme example of this is phantom limb pain. In this condition an amputee can feel severe pain in a limb that is no longer there. How is this possible? Because the nerves are still reporting pain messages as if they were coming from the vanished limb. In your brain, you still feel pain and that pain is as real as when you had your damaged limb.

Let's continue and investigate exactly how a pain system can malfunction, and how you can use this knowledge to successfully make the journey out of pain.

Meet the Enemy Within...

To understand how your pain system malfunctions, I'm going to tell you *'The Terrible Tale of When I Smashed My Thumb'*.

It went like this...

I was working with my son Benjamin to put a ceiling in my garage (a task I had successfully put off for twenty-five years). It was the end of a long day and all I had to do was hammer in one more nail. It was in an awkward corner. So I gingerly held the nail, took a wild swipe at it with the hammer... and missed it completely. What I did do was smash my thumb.

At this point I would like to relate I remained as calm as a Hindu cow in a state of serenely mindful presence. The truth is that I yelled out something unprintable, dropped my hammer (just as well there was no one below me) and wobbled down the ladder so I could curl up in a corner and moan.

That's what happened on the outside. Inside my body, something complex and marvellous was going on. When I first hit my thumb I stimulated three types of nerves. First was an A-beta nerve fibre which carries messages extremely fast. The message I got through this fibre was that something had touched the outside of my thumb – very (*very*) firmly. This first message was carried straight up my arm to the nerves in my spinal column, and then to my brain.

This was followed almost immediately by a message from my A-delta nerve fibre. The A-delta fibre is smaller and slightly slower. This second message was interpreted in my brain as a sharp intense pain (that's when I yelled and dropped my hammer).

The third and final message was from the C fibre. This fibre acts more slowly than the other two. It transmitted a deep, nauseating ache about two seconds after the blow. This is the part where I stumbled down the ladder to look for a corner in which to assume the foetal position.

But by the time I reached the floor, I noticed the pain was changing again. When I looked down at my thumb, I saw a vague bluish tinge underneath the nail. Already my thumb looked swollen, red, and felt hot.. My thumb began to throb. This was the start of a process called peripheral sensitisation.

The blue colour under my nail meant that blood vessels in the area had been broken and I was getting a bruise (or haematoma). As the blood under my nail started to clot, it released chemotactic factors, which are a call to arms for your immune system. They began the inflammatory process.

My C fibres (which had caused the deep aching pain) started to produce a group of substances known as the inflammatory soup. This 'soup' includes substance P, bradykinin, and others with long Latin names. These caused blood vessels in the area to further dilate – increasing the hot redness. All the substances in this inflammatory soup are algogenic, meaning they induce pain.

This inflammatory process is again part of what keeps you safe. The substances released into my thumb – the same ones making it sore and red and hot – are essential to the healing process.

I went inside and started looking for a painkiller. I now work as a pain specialist and used to be a family doctor, so as you might expect, I could not find even the simplest pain med in the whole house. I therefore resorted to the good old fashioned anaesthetics of our civilisation – alcohol and television. I poured a good slug of whiskey and sat down to watch some TV pulp to try and take my mind off my throbbing thumb. The whiskey worked a bit; the TV didn't.

And then something fascinating started to happen. Over the next hour I became aware that the pain from my thumb extended up my forearm to my elbow. It was now 11pm, so I went to bed. I tossed and turned, trying to get to sleep. At this stage the pain reached all the way up to my neck, the left side of my head, and across my shoulder and chest.

This was a different pain from my initial swollen thumb. It was not a throbbing pain, but an intense burning pain. And I was sweaty, grumpy, exhausted and nauseous.

The question was: what on earth was going on?

I smacked my thumb with a hammer, and now I have a weird burning pain extending all the way up my arm into my neck? I thought to myself: *This is not normal.*

And I was quite right. A process was taking place that occurs for everyone in chronic pain. And it's one of the main drivers of any pain that lasts longer than three months.

Here's what was REALLY happening.

Dodgy Don and the Pain Amplifier...

As the hammer struck my thumb a message was sent along my nerves. At this point, it was just a message and had no intrinsic meaning. It's the same as putting your ear to a telephone line and trying to interpret the signal. Until it's decoded at the other end you won't be able to understand the conversation.

The message decoding happens in your brain. But first (and this is important) the message has to pass through **two** different nervous systems (think of them as communication networks). These are the **peripheral nervous system (1)** and the **central nervous system (2)**.

When I smashed my thumb, the pain message started in the little nerve endings there, and was then transmitted down the nerves in my arm. It travelled via the peripheral system. Then the message **reached the spinal cord (3)**. This is where the peripheral system ends and the message needs to be transmitted to the central nervous system, which resides in the spinal cord and brain.

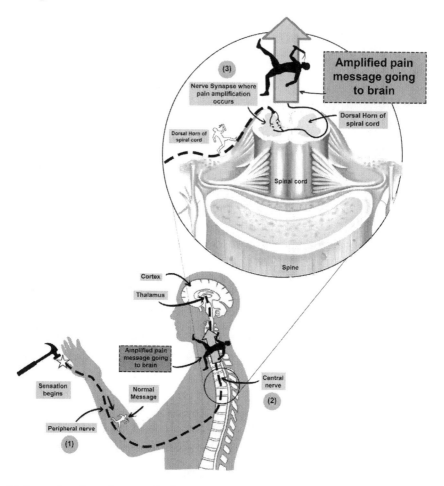

This point is where all the magic (and mischief) happens. For the message to go from the peripheral nervous system to the central nervous system, one nerve ending needs to talk to the other.

I don't know about you, but when I was a kid we used to play a game called telephone whispers. It works like this: a group of kids sit in a line, and one kid whispers a message in the ear of the other. The next kid whispers what they thought they heard, and the message goes along the line. And, no surprise, by the time the message reaches the kid at the end it has morphed into something completely different.

This is what happens to the message going from the area of pain – in this case my thumb – up to my brain. When the nerve carrying the pain message reaches the spinal cord there are several receptors waiting to receive the message.

Let us do a thought experiment together. In our thought experiment there is a tiny man (let's call him Arthur) standing on the nerve in my thumb, waiting for the nerve ending to give him a message. As the hammer hit my thumb, the message is handed to Arthur, who whirls around and runs as fast as he can along the nerve. He screeches to a halt at the end of the nerve **(1)**, puffing slightly and then is faced by a chasm at the **synapse (2)** – the point where one nerve system feeds into the other.

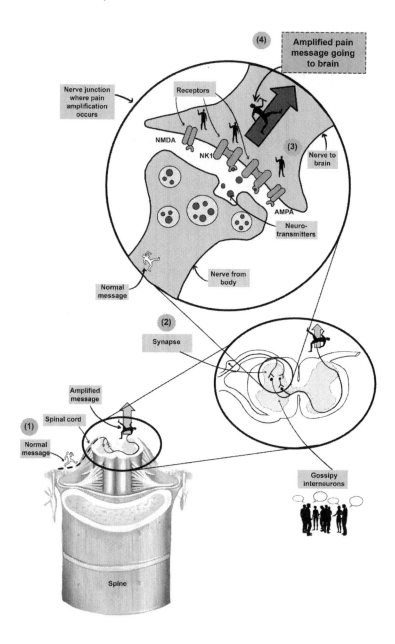

This is the point where the peripheral nervous system stops and now needs to talk to the central nervous system, starting in the spinal cord. Arthur can't cross the chasm of the synapse, so this is where he has to pass the message on. But, across the chasm, Arthur is faced by not one, but a group of people.

Arthur has to choose who he's going to pass it to. He has to choose between Straight Sam, Dodgy Don, and Tricky Trudy. If he hands the message over to the Straight Sam, who lives in the solidly built **AMPA receptor (3)** – Sam will collect the message and faithfully continue up to the brain. The message that reaches the brain will be exactly the same message that Arthur picked up at my thumb.

However, Arthur is dazzled by Dodgy Don in the glossy NMDA receptor. He throws the message over to Don, and as Don receives it something sinister happens. As Don whirls around to continue up the spinal cord, he takes the message and stretches it into a completely different shape.

So now, the message that reaches the brain is not the same as the one that started in the thumb **(4)**. It is much larger, and distorted. Your brain can only decipher the final message it receives, and assumes that message is an accurate representation of the state of your body. Your brain does not know that the pain message has been altered by Dodgy Don. So you may feel terrible pain, even though in reality minimal damage has been done.

Therefore, I thumped my thumb with the hammer. And a few hours later, lying in bed, I have pain that's magnified far beyond what it should be if I was receiving accurate pain messages.

What you're hearing here is laying the foundation for a profound insight. When you realise that the pain you feel is not always an accurate representation of what is going on in your body, it changes your relationship with chronic pain completely.

As I lay there at 2am, my whole upper right side on fire with a strange burning nerve pain, I reflected on what was happening. I was experiencing what is known as amplified pain or pain sensitisation.

The Gossips in Your Spinal Cord

If you look at how my pain spread, it highlights another aspect of amplified pain. Our sensory system is divided into segments. All the information from a particular part of your body enters a designated segment of the spinal cord and nowhere else. For example, all the information from my thumb and index finger comes into the sixth neck segment. All the information from my middle finger comes into the seventh neck segment, and so on.

In this picture you can see the C6 segment that covers my thumb and then extends up my arm to my spine (1). At the synapse where Straight Sam, Dodgy Don and Tricky Trudy wait, there are also a group of tiny, short nerves – Gossipy Gerty and her friends – also known as the interneurons (2). Gerty is a very important interneuron known as a WDR – wide dynamic range cell. In other words, she can gossip with any other nerves that come into her circle. She is the greatest gossip of all, picking up all manner of nerve signals from the body and transmitting them a few millimetres up and down the spinal cord to her other gossipy friends.

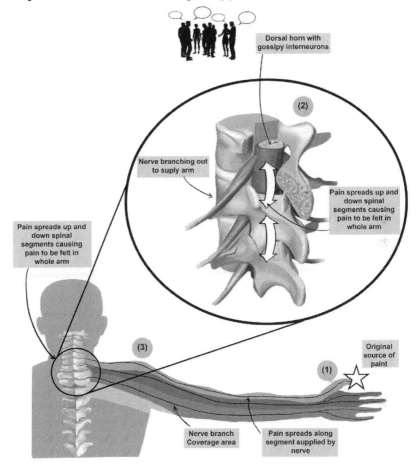

Trying to get to sleep that night, I imagined Gerty and her friends talking to each other, saying things like, "You'll never believe what happened in the thumb. I heard it was REALLY bad."

And then Gerty saying: "Yes, well you know what I'm going to do? I'm going to tell my friend Edna, a WDR cell in the segment above us about this – she really ought to know." And so my pain spread up into my neck and shoulder **(3)**. And then: "Well, you know, Bertha the WDR who lives down a segment has no idea what's going on, and I heard it really was a Big Deal." And so the pain spread down through the rest of my arm and into my chest.

As these gossipy nerve cells spread the news, the segments above and below them in the spinal cord get activated as well. They pick up the distorted and amplified pain message and transmit it back to the brain. As each segment is turned on, the pain message spreads and you feel pain in a wider area.

Again, your brain only receives the last message in this chain of communication. And if this last message is coming from all the activated segments, your brain accepts this, and (as with me) your pain now affects a much larger area. This is process called expansion of the receptor field.

Your brain receives this giant message of pain from your nerves, and has no way to stop and say, "Hey, wait a minute. You say the thumb got mashed. Well and good, but what's all this about pain in the *shoulder*? What's *that* got to do with it?"

Like a trusting newscaster, your brain believes everything the nerves tell it, and now you have widespread pain. Or, in my case, I had an awful burning pain covering a quarter of my body, and all I'd done was hit my thumb.

Which brings us to the last piece of the puzzle. For anyone who's hit their thumb before (you have my sympathies) you would know this is not a normal reaction. But it happened, because in my case, there were other factors at play.

I mentioned before how I felt awful – sweaty, grumpy, heart racing. This is part of what's known as a fight or flight response. It's an important evolutionary survival response we all have. We see something dangerous – like a charging bull – and our system goes into overdrive. We're flooded with adrenaline, our heart pounds, our muscles are filled with oxygen-rich blood. Between one moment and the next we are ready to run top speed away from the danger... or make a desperate stand and fight it off.

For some reason, after hitting my thumb, I had a massive fight or flight response. Lying there at 2am trying to get to sleep, this inappropriate survival mechanism was also amping up my pain and making my life even more miserable.

Why did I have such a reaction?

The Caveman Brain

When you have an injury, the physical damage is not the only ingredient in how much pain you feel.

When a pain message comes up to your brain it goes to the midbrain – the thalamus. The thalamus is like the switching station of the brain. Messages come from all over the body and the thalamus decides if they're important or not, and sends them on to various other parts of the brain.

The midbrain is a fascinating area. It's a primal part of the brain, and one that we share with all other mammals. Its main task is to ensure our survival. Because of this it's more likely to over-respond to threats, particularly if they're similar to other threats we've faced in the past.

Back in the caveman days, if you saw a rustle in the grass, it could either be a dangerous predator or just a harmless breeze. Our great-great-great-ancestors had three choices when confronted with a possible threat. They could run, fight, or do nothing.

If they got it wrong nine times out of ten, and the rustle in the grass was nothing – no big deal. But if they got it wrong once, and the rustle of leaves was in fact a Sabertooth Tiger getting ready for the final attack, then they were lunch.

So we – the caveman survivors, the ones who didn't end up on the menu – survived in part because our midbrain overreacts to possible threats. It will trigger a fight or flight response first, and then verify if we really needed to get the surge of adrenaline, heart-thumping rush of fear, and leap back ten feet.

In my case, my midbrain decided my thumb was under attack. I needed to escape. This triggered an autonomic response. My heart rate went up, my breathing increased (setting off hyperventilation) and I was in a cold sweat. I was ready and primed to run top speed away from my attacker. The only problem with this otherwise excellent strategy? My thumb was quite securely attached to my body. I could not escape the pain. The fight or flight response only served to make me feel worse.

This is the next manifestation of amplified pain, and now we are getting to the crux of the matter.

Why did this process turn on in the first place? Not everyone who smacks their thumb can't sleep at 2am because their whole arm and shoulder is on fire.

The reason I had such an extreme reaction has to do with history. Eighteen years ago when I crashed my hang glider at fifty miles an hour, smacking into it shoulder first, the impact ripped down into my back.

Following my crash I had seven years of chronic pain. The first impact had been my shoulder on that same side. You had better believe my pain system took this new injury seriously.

My survival instincts leapt into action because my pain system was already primed. In the years after my crash I had learned everything I needed to know about how to amplify pain. For years I had (unknowingly) reinforced pain pathways that were now thankfully dormant.

But reviving old neural pathways is just like riding a bike. You may not ride a bike for eighteen years, but hop on one and you'll find you can still pedal your way down the road. The neural pathways laid down when you learned to ride a bike are still there, ready to be switched on. And similarly the neural pathways from my hang gliding crash and the years of pain that followed were still there, like old circuitry just waiting to be turned on.

Let's repaint the scenario.

When I smacked my thumb, Dodgy Don took the amplified pain message up to my brain. In the thalamus he hands it over to Homer, the switchboard operator who receives it and has a look.

"Ok, says here we just smashed our thumb." Homer, sitting in his office, scratches his head. There're tons of messages coming in all the time, but this is a red PAIN message – so it might be important.

He picks up the phone and dials the big boss John at the head office – the anterior cingulate cortex (ACC) – otherwise known as the prefrontal cortex. This is where memory and emotion live.

"Hey boss, says here we just got our thumb smashed. What do you reckon?"

"Hang on a minute," snaps John. He rifles around in some filing cabinets. "Ah, here we go." There's silence on the other end of the line.

"Boss? What's up?"

"Well... let's see. I remember we damaged the arm and shoulder on that side in a hang gliding accident. We were in awful pain for years. So yup, you were right to call me, Homer. This is VERY important." And then the key words:

"We had better keep a very careful eye on this!"

John slams down the phone. Turning in his chair he flicks some switches. Lights blink on and all systems are go. He's just turned the nerves coming from that area up to maximum sensitivity. Then he pushes The Red Button. Sirens start wailing and a big voice booms out, 'Fight and Flight everyone!' The ladies in the limbic system open the adrenaline valves, and it's all on.

So all pain messages from my arm are amplified. Added to that, Gerty and her friends have spread the pain message. And now my autonomic system is in full fight and flight mode.

It's a nightmare scenario. And for many people, variations on this process are happening 24/7. Sadly, they and their doctors continue to blame this on 'a bad back' or 'a busted shoulder', and ignore the real cause

*

Now you understand how amplified pain works. It is an incredibly important part of chronic pain. Every day people come to my clinic whose pain started years ago. It could have been from a small accident, or a serious accident, or from nothing at all. They've had many investigations and no one can find the true cause of their pain.

The truth is this: their original injury healed long ago but their pain system is still stuck on red alert. It is amplifying all messages coming from that area up to the level of pain. Also, because of the gossipy interneurons, the pain has spread to a much larger area than the original injury. This process has no timeframe. It can continue full force for the rest of your life unless you do something about it.

Deeply understanding this process is the first and most important step. I strongly suggest you read this chapter as many times as it takes for you to really understand what goes on between Arthur, Gerty, John, and all the rest. It is completely central to why you are still in pain, and how you're going to get better. If you are a more visual person, you can go to www.6KeysPainFree.com to watch a video of this process.

The rest of this book will deal with what you can do with this knowledge. By the end of it you'll know the Six Keys to follow to retake control of your pain system and get back in the driver's seat of your life.

Action Steps:

1. Do you deeply understand amplified pain?
2. Think. How could this knowledge apply to your pain?
3. For the next few days, carry a notepad around with you. Every time you feel your habitual pain, write down 3 things:
   - What do you think caused the pain?
   - What thought runs through your mind when you feel the pain?
   - What emotion do you feel?

This trains a very important part of your brain, which we are going to further explore in the treatment section.

3
The Three
Chronic Pain Types

Now you understand amplified pain, we're going to go a little deeper into how this works. Over the last fourteen years of running my pain clinic, I've noticed there are three basic chronic pain 'types'. Although you may have characteristics of all three, I've noticed that generally one type will be dominant.

In the next three chapters we're going to explore what these types are and how they work. And then we'll get to the exciting part – how to treat them.

There are some insights that go deep into the roots of chronic pain and apply to every pain type. And there are some basic principles of practice that will help you no matter which pain type you are. However, for each pain type there's an optimal course of treatment.

The three pain types are:

Reactive, Hotline, and Autonomic.
These pain types represent the ways in which your body and mind reacts to being in chronic pain. Once you identify your type and understand it, a lot of what's been happening so far with your pain will become clear. Things that have puzzled

the many doctors and specialists you've been to see will now make sense, and you'll have a plan for getting out of chronic pain.

I encourage you to read up on all three types and understand them fully before you decide which is your primary pain type. You may find you have elements from one or two types, but identifying your dominant type will tell you where to start and what treatment course to take.

Before we get onto the three types however, let's review what you've learned so far:
- You can get pain – sometimes excruciating pain – when there's very little or no physical damage in your body. This is known as amplified pain or pain sensitisation.
- Your pain expands to cover a much larger area than was damaged.

It's this disconnect between pain and physical damage that leads to so many unnecessary treatments and surgery.

Here's a quick summary of the three types before we go into more detail. See if you can recognise your pain in any of them.

Hotline Pain

This is when your pain is unpredictable. It can be burning, tingling, shooting, aching, or any combination of these. It can move around – going from one part of your body to the other. It has no obvious pattern, and can attack without warning. The sheer unpredictability of this pain can be one of its most distressing characteristics. Hotline pain can also cause 'weird' sensations that aren't exactly pain, but can't easily be explained, leading some people to doubt their sanity as well as their body. In some rare cases, Hotline pain is simply constantly there.

Reactive Pain

This kind of pain appears to make sense. People with Reactive pain know (more or less) what will cause it to come on, and how long it usually lasts. The pain patterns are quite specific for each individual. Reactive pain can be caused by certain activities, like walking or sitting too long, or it can be worse at certain times of day, or in particular environments. However, while this pain appears to make sense, and people with it accept their explanation, there's actually something quite different going on. We'll explore this in the Reactive pain chapter.

Autonomic Pain

Autonomic pain is amplified by stress, and in turn this type of pain affects the rest of your body in some unexpected ways. People with Autonomic pain can also suffer from a raft of other symptoms like: irritable bowel syndrome, hot and cold flushes, dizziness, heart palpitations, irritable bladder, shortness of breath, and more. These are the manifestation of an over-reactive fight and flight system. In most cases, people don't see the connection between the pain they're feeling and these other equally distressing health problems. But they are closely connected, and treating them together makes all the difference.

In all three types, the mechanism causing the pain is the same: amplification of the pain message by your malfunctioning pain system. But they present in different ways, and need to be treated differently.

Now you have the overview, it's time to explore the first of the chronic pain types.

TYPE #1: HOTLINE

Hotline pain is the purest example of amplified pain. It occurs at the point (known as the nerve synapse) where your peripheral nervous system talks to your central nervous system. This is where Arthur met Dodgy Don in the previous chapter.

In Hotline pain, this connection is unstable. Your body has made a 'hotline' from the painful area up to your brain. However, there is one more interesting variation here: the amplification may be quite changeable. It may not only alter the volume of the pain, it may also shift around your pain system and cause pain to appear in other parts of your body.

The Hotline process can also change the characteristic of the message. This changes the type of pain that you feel in an area. For people with Hotline pain, it is almost as if there is a little sprite running up and down your pain system turning the amplifiers on and off at a whim. This can be infinitely frustrating.

Here are the characteristics of the Hotline pain type:

- The pain can be constantly present in some form, although it can change in character.
- The pain can be aching, burning, stabbing, prickling, shooting, tearing, and it can change from one type to the other without rhyme or reason.
- The pain can shift around in a weird and unpredictable way.
- It can go from mild to incredibly intense with no warning.
- The pain is not tied to any particular activity or time of day.

As the pain is caused by nerves behaving badly, anything can happen. The pain can be very distressing due to its unpredictability.

Hotline pain can also include 'weird' sensations. I've had people tell me the part of their body that hurts feels different from the rest of their body. Or they encounter strange sensations like water running on their skin, or an insect crawling across their back. The point is that with Hotline pain the neurotransmitters are not just amplifying the pain, they're distorting it too. So unusual and 'weird' sensations can be part and parcel of this type of pain. The medical name for this is neuropathic pain.

With Hotline pain, you're never sure when it's going to come on and be horribly sore, or where it will go next. I've even had people come to see me with pain that started on one side of their body, then shifted to the other side with no obvious explanation.

I recently saw Carol, who has had pain for a number of years. She described the pain in terms of lightning. She said at times it felt like sheet lightning and at other times it felt like forked lightning, while there were times it felt 'like thunder'. The pain would move over her body. She was never able to predict where it would come but almost every day it was there and it was very distressing.

She also never knew how severe it was going to be. She described her life as living in a cage where somebody else had control of the lighting, the temperature, the flow of air, and everything to do with her life.

The essence of this pain and the thing that got to her the most was that it truly did not make sense. And because of that she had lost her feeling of being in control of her life and had become virtually housebound.

One thing she did note was that whenever her husband suggested they go on a holiday or an outing, the night before they were due to go, her pain would become much more severe.

She would then have to take to her bed once again. She realised that in some way a part of her was sabotaging any chance of her enjoying life. Carol had seen many doctors, psychiatrists, alternative practitioners, and tried all sorts of medication. Unfortunately, none of the experts had made any difference and the medications either didn't work or gave her nasty side effects. So far, nobody had been able to explain her pain to her in a way that made sense.

Having looked at how pain amplification occurs and how Hotline pain works, you can see she had a classic example of a Hotline malfunction. The pre-holiday, unconscious self-sabotage she experienced was also quite common, and this can take many shapes. We will be exploring why this happens later in the book, and what you can do to dismantle it.

Carol and I discussed how amplified pain works. Just this knowledge changed her from a victim to somebody who now understood. This was the first step on her journey out of chronic pain. She then mastered the Six Keys, which included mind-body techniques [1,2,3] that we will be exploring together later in the book (chapter 7).

Carol found a few techniques that worked wonderfully well for her, and over a number of months her pain lessened and became much more manageable. She was also able to influence the self-sabotage to the extent that she and her husband successfully went away for a weekend. This was a huge step, and she said it was the beginning of getting her life back.

She has continued to manage her pain, which has not gone away completely but is no longer the centre of her life. She is a new lady. Truly knowledge is power.

I remember Annette, whom I saw a number of months ago. I always spend a long time exploring a new patient's history. Annette stated that she always edited her story, because she was embarrassed to describe her complex myriad of symptoms. She had pain that affected mainly the lower half of her body, and it had so many different faces. It could feel like her tissues were ripping apart, a shooting or burning pain, and many more variations.

But the thing that concerned her most was that she would get weird sensations. At times she felt like there was water running down her side and she would look down expecting her trouser leg to be wet. There were times where she would swear there was an insect crawling over her skin, or more distressing, a worm crawling under her skin. And then the sensations would go as strangely as they had come.

She had seen a neurologist who was as puzzled as she, and in his letter he could not explain these weird sensory changes in an otherwise normally-functioning person. When I examined her I found, just as the neurologist did, that there were no obvious signs of damage in her neurological system. What she had instead was a <u>malfunction</u>.

You see the sensory system is capable of infinite variations in function. Not only can the different receptors amplify or shrink messages, they can also change their nature. Therefore what starts off as a feeling of slight warmth may be changed into unbearable heat or can be twisted by your sensory system into a message of something crawling under your skin.

The message, when it reaches your brain, is real but it is not an accurate representation of what is really happening in your body. You are not going nuts, it is just your pain system malfunctioning.

Understanding this gave Annette great freedom and set her mind at ease. We then explored mind-body techniques [1,2,3] and she was slowly able to return her badly-behaved pain system to a more normal function. The key lies in understanding.

How Pain Medication Fits Into this Picture

Hotline pain can be difficult to settle down. It is here that I find judicious use of certain medications can be useful.

My view on medication is that it is just another tool in your toolbox that you can use to manage your pain. Often people rely too much on, and expect too much from medication – especially in the treatment of chronic pain.

At best, most medications will reduce pain by a maximum of 30 to 50%, and if this is what happens, you are doing wonderfully well. Unfortunately, every medication comes with a list of side effects, and at the end of the day you need to balance the risk and the benefits of each medication.

So it is a tool that can help you get to the point where you are able to apply other techniques including mind-body techniques, exercise, trigger points, natural movement – all of which have no side effects. As you get better at these techniques, their benefit becomes greater. In fact there really are no limits to how much help you can get when you apply your mind to a problem that in most cases is primarily a malfunction of your nervous system.

I view human beings as a mind with the body attached – the mind is the boss. If you use your mind with knowledge and understanding, it can be the most powerful tool to break out of the prison of chronic pain and live a fully productive and joyous life.

The easy thing about medication is that you just put it in your mouth and it will do its job. This is a double-edged sword in that you may come to rely on the medication with minimal input from yourself. However, when used appropriately, it can be literally a lifesaver.

From a medical point of view, Hotline pain is a subgroup of neuropathic pain. This means that the pain arises from a malfunction in your nervous system. This is recognised to be particularly difficult to treat with most commonly-used pain medications [4,5].

However there are a number of medications that can be quite effective in reducing the irritability and the irrational behaviour of your nervous system. Some have been around for many years while others are the new kids on the block.

The most commonly used are low-dose Tricyclic antidepressants like Amitriptyline and Nortriptyline. These have been around since the 1960s. They work by blocking neurotransmitters. Neurotransmitters are substances that transport messages between nerves which, as you remember, are where the initial amplification of pain messages occur.

Going back to chapter 2, the neurotransmitter carries the message from Arthur to Dodgy Don as he throws it across the synapse chasm.

Tricyclic antidepressants affect mainly the transmitter called norepinephrine. They also have other complex effects on NMDA receptors and your autonomic nervous system [6,7] and therefore help sleep, relaxation, and irritable bowel/bladder.

As with all medications, there are many side effects, which often limit their usefulness.

There are also newer antidepressant medications that change the function of your brain and nervous system by blocking both serotonin and norepinephrine uptake. These are the main neurotransmitters in the nervous system, and this increases their levels in the body. This reduces anxiety and depression and will also reduce your pain. These include Venlafaxine, Duloxetine and Milnacipran [8,9] .

Another potentially useful group include certain antiepileptic drugs. These drugs work by stabilising the membrane that sheaths nerves. Nerve membranes are fascinating. They are punctured by little holes, and within these holes there is a tiny pump that pushes charged particles from one side of the membrane to another. When the concentration reaches a certain threshold, the nerve will fire. If you are able to stabilise or reduce the activity of the pump, then the irritability of the membrane is reduced and the nerve will not fire as easily. It simmers down and you feel less neuropathic pain.

This is how antiepileptic drugs will quieten the little sprite that is wreaking havoc with your pain amplifiers. These medications include Gabapentin and Pregabalin and are being used successfully by millions of people around the world.

Information on medication is constantly changing, so check www.6KeysPainFree.com for the latest data.

If you feel like your pain just doesn't make sense, or if it is there all the time, you need to look seriously at the Hotline pain type.

Action Steps

1. If you feel like Hotline pain matches what you have, we still recommend you read the other two types because often there is some overlap. Once you have truly understood this knowledge, you will have mastered the First Key.

2. After you've done this, go to chapter 7 and begin to learn about and practice the mind-body techniques recommended for Hotline pain.

4

Reactive Pain

'The ability to ask the right question is more than half the battle of finding the right answer.'
- Thomas J Watson

So far we've looked at the Hotline pain type and how this works. But this is not how everyone experiences chronic pain. The next type we're going to look at is the Reactive pain type.

This is a fascinating type, and is what I experienced when I had back pain for seven years. To learn about the Reactive pain type, we're going to return to where we had left the story of my hang-gliding crash in chapter 1 – with my realisation that I didn't have pain at work.

The Pain That Only Happened Outside Work

After my hang-gliding crash I continued struggling with significant pain for seven years. It only took me a mere seven years to ask the question: "Why do I not have much pain at work?"

And at first, I didn't look at this fact too closely. I was busy running around chasing my tail (as we all do).

But then one day I stopped and thought, Wow, that is weird.

I then tried to justify the question away. Well, I don't get pain because at work I'm really busy. (This was true.) Or: I don't do the same physical activities at work as at home. (Which was actually not true – they were very similar.)

But the question kept coming back. So I examined it in more detail, and the more I thought about it, the more odd it seemed.

When I reflected on the situation, I did all the same things at work – sitting, walking turning, lifting – as I did in a normal day at home on the weekend. Yet at work I hardly felt any pain, while at home I was frequently hobbling and groaning with excruciating stabs and aches in my back.

It turns out that what I had was the Reactive pain type. We'll be going into some of the other common Reactive patterns, but first I would like you to see how this insight was hiding from me in plain sight all these years.

I was able to ignore this fact for the same reason you may be ignoring the hidden truth about your pain – because we are all explanation-making machines. We feel pain, we think, *Why is this?* and then we create an explanation that makes sense at first glance. Once we have an acceptable explanation, we stop searching.

Let's go one level deeper into my Reactive pain pattern.

In the morning I would lie in bed and mentally prepare myself for getting up. I needed to do this because as I made the first movement, I would get an agonising 10 out of 10 pain in my lower back.

The pain would start in my lower back and shoot down my leg. I would break into a cold sweat, knowing I had to get up for work, waiting for the next stab of pain as I slowly inched myself to the edge of the bed.

It would take me many minutes to get from my back to my side and roll out of bed. Then I'd shower, get ready for work, and my pain would slowly settle. This agonising drama repeated itself every morning for seven years.

I explained it to myself like this: Well, I've been lying down with gravity acting on me all night, and this must have done something to my back. And then I have to change position, and that sets off the awful pain. So when I get up I have to resettle my spine and that's why I have the pain.

When I started asking the question: "Why do I not have pain at work?" It made me re-examine everything, including this morning pain. The truth was that before I had my accident I'd been lying in bed and getting up in the morning with no pain. We are all designed to do this – it's completely natural.

So why, seven years after my injury, did I have this 10/10 pain every morning? Then, I remembered the first morning after my accident. I'd been drugged up on morphine through the night but now the opiates had worn off. I woke up, and the first time I went to move, that 10/10 pain hit. It's easy to see why. My shoulders were dislocated, my back had herniated discs, and everything was bruised, swollen, and traumatised.

It was a horrible twenty minutes, but eventually I got up, tottered off to the bathroom and somehow made it through the day. I went to bed that night exhausted. The next morning when I woke, just before I went to move, I remembered what had happened the previous day. I gritted my teeth and I had the same pain. That evening, as I got into bed, I thought, I wonder if I'm going to have the same pain in the morning?

And I did. And the next morning too. And on and on for the next seven years.

So the question is: what exactly was going on?

To answer this, we need to go back in time to the 1890s and meet the great Russian scientist Dr Ivan Pavlov, and his group of happy, hungry dogs in a very famous experiment.

Pavlov[1,2,3] created a device to measure how much saliva his dogs would produce. In the first stage of the experiment, he brought the dogs some food and they salivated. In the next stage, he entered the dogs' enclosure and rang a bell, and they didn't make saliva. Then, he brought the dogs food and rang the bell at the same time. They smelt the food, heard the bell, and produced saliva. Pavlov then repeated this several times.

The last stage was the most important. Pavlov entered the dogs' enclosure and just rang the bell. There was no food yet still the dogs made saliva.

With this experiment, Pavlov created a new connection in the dogs' minds and bodies. Before he did this experiment, no dog had ever salivated when a bell rang. They would only do this in the presence of food. With a few simple steps Pavlov connected an unconscious reaction in the dogs' bodies (making saliva) to a new external stimulus (the bell ringing).

This was Pavlov's genius insight. He called it a conditioned response. What happened in this experiment will explain what happened to me each morning, and what is happening for so many of you in the Reactive pain type.

Each morning as I went to move for the first time, this was the specific external stimulus. The first time I had the 10/10 pain there was an obvious cause for it – my back was badly damaged. But in the months following my crash, the tear in my disc and the swelling around the vertebrae slowly reduced. Seven years later, my back had completely healed but the pattern continued.

Here is what was happening: as I woke, my brain recognised the conditions were correct to run its program. It then switched on to full capacity all the amplifiers on the neural pathway from my back. As I first went to move, a nerve message would fire, and as it zoomed across to my spinal cord it would be amplified many times [4] (as you learned about in chapter 2). I would then feel an agonising 10/10 pain when the message arrived in my brain. This same program also turned on my fight and flight response, making me break into a cold, shaking sweat.

That first morning set the stage. And in my mind something important happened: I connected the pain and the external conditions. I thought, I hope this doesn't happen again....

But a small time bomb was already ticking away in my brain. Every morning as I woke, the conditions were the same and I ran the same pain program. The external stimulus was the same and my pain system would produce the pain.

Like Pavlov ringing the bell as he delivered food, I was connecting my awful back pain with getting out of bed. After this had happened enough times I expected it with total conviction and it became inevitable.

*

Right now, you're all probably thinking, yes but….

"Yes, this is an interesting story, but my pain isn't like that."

"Yes, but I get pain when I sit, and I get it worse when I'm at work."

"Yes, but my pain turns on when I stand or walk for too long. And it's because my MRI shows I have disc damage."

Or, "Yes, but I've had surgery."

"I have spondylosis…" "Scoliosis…" "Spinal Stenosis… rotator cuff tears… osteoarthritis in my knee/hip… so this doesn't apply to me?"

In short, you're probably thinking, yes, but my pain is different from this AND I've been given a diagnosed cause, so this obviously isn't happening to me.

The 'Yes, but...' explanation may have come from your own observation or you may have been given this by an expert – complete with MRIs, x-rays and other scans. Perhaps this explanation has satisfied you so far because on the surface it makes sense, just like mine did.

So let's dig a little deeper.

If I showed you ten other people with almost identical MRI pictures and back pain (for example), you would note two very interesting things. First, their pain would come on during completely different activities; some would have more pain when sitting, some when standing.

Some would have pain at night, others in the morning. Some would get pain when they walked for too long, and some would have pain from specific activities like gardening or cycling.

And second, each person would have a well thought-out and plausible reason for why their pain came on when it did. Their explanation would have a certain symmetry to it (otherwise known as circular reasoning). "I get pain when I sit for longer than forty minutes. Therefore sitting for longer than forty minutes causes my pain." Perfectly obvious, logical... and inaccurate.

If the diagnosed cause of pain was accurate, everyone with the same MRI (or other investigation) should have the same pain. And it should be caused by the exact same activities. In other words, the same mechanical stress on the structure should cause the same pain.

Let's compare the irregular behaviour of Reactive pain with pain that's caused by a mechanical problem – for example a broken leg. Every person with a fractured femur will experience pain when they put weight on it. The pain will lessen when they take weight off the leg and lie down.

But for Reactive pain this is plainly not the case. Which begs the question: how accurate then is *your* explanation for your pain?

People in the Reactive pain type have unconsciously created their pain patterns based on what happened when their pain first began. Unknowingly, they have paired an external stimulus with their pain. Over time, this means a pattern is created in their brain and their pain gets amplified whenever the external circumstances are right.

It becomes like running a program. When conditions are right, you fire up the program and neural patterns laid down over weeks, months and years activate, making pain inevitable.

*

Here are some examples of Reactive pain patterns I've encountered over the years in my pain clinic.

The first one is delayed pain. This is usually introduced to me by someone saying: "When I do a particular activity I really enjoy, I'm ok, but I know I'm going to pay for it later."

John was a keen and accomplished tennis player. He was in his late-30s. Tennis played a huge part in his life – it kept him fit, he loved the competition (especially winning), and his wife plus most of his friends were tennis players. He played mainly on the weekend.

He had decided to give up his beloved tennis. He was supremely frustrated. The reason he gave was that for the last three years he had almost no pain whilst he played, but he would then "pay for it" with the most excruciating low back, buttock and leg pain two days later. This was usually Monday or Tuesday and this pain took most of the rest of the week to settle – just in time for his next tennis game. The pain interfered significantly with his ability to work. He had seen a back specialist and his MRI was completely normal. He had had treatment from various practitioners with very little benefit.

John's story is typical of a subtype of Reactive pain pattern. The pain comes on usually two to three days after doing the specific activity. Whether it's walking for a long time, gardening, playing tennis – whatever it is – Reactive pain sufferers know without doubt the pain will turn on later. They know this because it's happened every time for years. And the pain may then linger for days.

Let's unpack the delayed pain pattern. For starters, there is no physiological reason why pain would switch on two to three days after an activity. If you injure an area while doing something, you will feel the pain right then and there. We know that pain messages will normally reach your brain in less than a second.

Sometimes an injury may set off inflammation that may take a few hours to start, but that's not two or three days. Finally, there is a condition called DOMS [6] (Delayed Onset Muscle Soreness.) This occurs when you do unaccustomed intense exercise. In this case you will notice the pain after twenty-four hours and it's a very specific 'sore muscle' kind of pain. It would feel different from your original injury or normal pain, and when you press the muscles they will be tender to the touch. Resting eases this pain, using the muscles makes it worse. It only occurs once or twice before the muscles 'harden' and accommodate to the new level of exercise. It is never a recurrent problem.

Apart from these easily-diagnosed causes of pain, there is no other physical explanation for pain that switches on a few days after a particular activity.

There is however, an explanation that makes perfect sense when you look at it from a different angle.

The first time they had significant pain, Reactive types thought, what on earth could have caused this pain? Ah yes, I went for a long walk two days ago, that must the reason I have pain now. Having made this connection, the question comes up the next time they go for walk: I wonder if it's going to hurt in two days' time? And the rest is history.

*

Another common pattern is the pain switching on at a particular time, often at night. Over the years I've met people who are regularly woken anywhere from midnight to five in the morning.

Wendy's pain woke her every morning at 3am, and then kept her awake for at least two hours.

Margot didn't have a set time when her pain came on, but it always woke her up five hours after she fell asleep.

Jack's pain came on at 11am every Monday, except public holidays when he didn't go into work.

When you look at this from a traditional medical perspective, it makes no sense. (Although in every case people had thought out their own explanation, which they had accepted for years.)

But when you realise the pain is being turned on by a conditioned response, the underlying cause of pain is crystal clear.

Here's how night pain works. You've injured your back, and at 3:07am you roll over, and something tweaks in your back. The pain wakes you, and with a groan you look at your cellphone. It's 3:07am. How awful.

You toss and turn and somehow fall back to sleep. When your alarm wakes you a few hours later you're exhausted. You get up and as you shower and get ready for work you remember the stab in your back woke you at 3:07. That's why you're so tired!

You struggle through the day, and at last make it home. Then, as you get ready for bed, the thought emerges: It was so awful being woken last night by the pain in my back, *I hope it doesn't happen again.*

And when it does, the next night you don't think: I hope it doesn't happen again. You think: Oh no! That awful pain is going to wake me in the early hours of the morning again. And it does.

We are habit-forming creatures. Habits are a vital part of how we learn and become functioning human beings. They're how you are able to drive, type, read – everything that's useful. But this habit mode doesn't discriminate whether the habit is helpful or harmful, it just turns on when conditions are right.

Unfortunately, people with this type of Reactive pain have unknowingly trained their pain system to turn on an amplified pain at a particular time of night, and unless they learn how to break this pattern it could continue for the rest of their life.

*

Another pattern is pain after sitting for a certain length of time. Sitting is an interesting one because today most adults spend more time sitting than any other time in history. And research shows this new mode isn't that good for you. Especially the way most people sit – hunched over their computers or steering wheels. It has been said "sitting is the new smoking". The recommended dose of sitting [7] is thirty minutes. After that, stand for a couple of minutes then start the next thirty minutes of sitting.

However, research aside, something different happens for people with Reactive pain and sitting. For starters, they get pain in different places.

Some people find sitting kills them in their shoulders, while others it's their upper back. For many it's their lower back. What is happening here is not that sitting is damaging their body, it's that they've unconsciously learnt to run a 'pain while sitting' program that will switch on after a certain length of time.

Sitting is not inherently a dangerous posture. It's a normal and natural position, as is standing, walking, bending and twisting. If we look at the physical side of sitting, the pressures in your back are slightly higher when you sit, but they are easily within safe tolerances.

People who can walk or jog (where there are bigger pressures in their back) should be able to sit quite comfortably. However, if you have a Reactive pain pattern connected with sitting, it can sometimes cause extreme pain.

Here's how it works: at some stage sitting (usually at work) with stress and prolonged time in a slumped position, your pain turns on. At this point, the pain may occur anywhere from your back to your shoulders, to your neck, to your buttocks.

The first time this happens, a little clock starts ticking in your head. So the next time before you sit down you have this little thought which goes:

Last time it hurt after I sat for this length of time... I wonder if it's going to hurt again?

The little clock starts ticking in your unconscious mind, and again you have pain while sitting. The third time the question is answered, and now you have an expectation of pain when you sit. You have now tied this external stimulus (sitting) to an unconscious response (pain amplification), and from now on you will have pain whenever you sit.

I have encountered people who have pain when they sit on hard chairs. I've also encountered people who have pain only when they sit on soft chairs. I've treated people who only have pain when they sit on car seats, or only have pain when they sit for more than twenty minutes etc.

To turn off this pain, using correct posture and having regular breaks is helpful. But the real issue is that whenever you sit you are loading a program that turns on your pain amplification, and that needs to be addressed for lasting pain relief.

*

The last Reactive pain pattern I've seen many times is the pain-free holiday. Here's an example:

Jennie came to see me very worried because she was about to embark on once-in-a-lifetime trip abroad with her husband. She was worried because she had chronic back pain and she was terrified this would flare up in a foreign country where she couldn't get the help she needed.

She was also worried about the pain ruining the trip she and her husband had been looking forward to for a long time. We discussed strategy, and I gave her some emergency medication to take with her and we booked a follow-up appointment for two weeks after she returned.

Two weeks after her return from Europe we met again.

"So, how was your holiday?" I asked.

"Wonderful," she beamed.

"And how was your back pain while you were away?"

"Fine, totally fine," she replied breezily. Then she frowned. "But... about a week after I got home it started again. So I'm wondering if you can do something for it."

"Ah." I leaned back in my chair. There was an opportunity opening up here, but it needed to be explored carefully. "So the whole time you were away – six weeks in all – you didn't have any pain?"

"Well, I had a little twinge here and there but nothing serious."

"And... do you think that's at all unusual?"

"No, not really."

"So why do you think your back pain went away when you were overseas?" I asked.

She thought for a minute. "Well... I guess I wasn't doing anything strenuous. I was relaxing."

Really? We talked some more and I got an accurate picture of her holiday. It became clear her holiday hadn't just involved sitting by a pool or on a beach. In fact, she'd been very active. She and her husband had journeyed through half of Europe. She'd walked every day, sometimes for hours. She'd trundled suitcases along cobbled streets. She'd contended with the stress of new languages, mad taxi drivers and long hours in buses and trains.

In fact, compared to her normal routine, the holiday abroad had been a real exertion.

So why hadn't her back played up and been painful?

I've seen this pattern often enough to offer an explanation. While she was abroad, Jennie was removed from all her normal environments. None of her usual triggers were there – those same triggers which cued her pain.

And so although she had demanded much more of her back than usual, she'd been mostly free of pain.

I explained how Reactive pain worked, and she left my consult room with a light in her eye and a determination to her step that boded well. And when I caught up with her again a couple of months later, her pain had gone – completely. It now behaved just like when she was on holiday. We're going to explore exactly what she did in later chapters.

*

Treating the Reactive pain type is interesting. It's the one I have personal experience with, and I've seen many people do extremely well once they recognise it.

The first and most vital step is recognising your pain pattern. Once you've found the external stimulus that turns on your conditioned pain response, the question arises: Ok, so... how do I switch it off?

Recognition in itself can sometimes be enough. For quite a few of my patients that's all it took. It's like blowing the cover of a confidence trickster, or calling your opponent's bluff in a game of poker. It takes courage and insight, but for many people the moment they do this everything changes and it is 'game over'.

I know this for a fact because a few months after I had my insight, I was able to wake and get out of bed with zero pain. And I still do that today many years later. However, other people need a more structured process, and we will now discuss this in detail.

The first step is to set up a court of enquiry inside your head or, if it works better for you, on a piece of paper. There is the prosecutor, the defence council, and the judge. They are all part of your mind, but each has their clearly appointed task. You can imagine them as vividly as you need to.

Here is a court case scenario I helped a patient of mine, Tom, visualise:

The inner judge pounds his gavel on the desk and calls order to the court. He announces: "We are hearing the case of a Tom, a 55-year-old man who has had good health up till now. His history is of a sharp, stabbing (at times burning) pain that appears in his neck and right shoulder. This comes on about twenty minutes after he sits down in front of his computer at work.

"It then rapidly becomes so intense that he has to stop and stretch. He takes a pain-killer then struggles through the day. It takes the night and most of the weekend to recover. His life is being ruined."

The defence will start and present its arguments:

"Three years ago our client was involved in a motor vehicle accident. He sustained a whiplash injury to his neck and has had ongoing significant pain from this injury.

"This is why we think our client still suffers pain from the injury:

1. We know that whiplash can cause chronic neck pain, which refers into the shoulder area.

2. His x-ray shows mild wear and tear with some disc narrowing and bony overgrowth in his lower neck and this is clearly evidence of damage. This has been confirmed by his chiropractor.

3. We also know that using a word processor, especially the mouse, can cause neck and shoulder pain which can be difficult to treat successfully.

"So your honour (addressing his inner judge), it is clear Tom injured his lower neck in a car crash, and this is causing his ongoing pain despite treatment."

With a nod, the judge continues. "The prosecutor will present his arguments."

"Thank you, your honour. Three years ago, Tom was involved in a minor motor vehicle accident where he bumped into a car in a parking lot. However, the pain actually came on a couple of days later at work. He thought back and assumed he had injured his neck during the accident, and now believes this is why he lives with pain. However, these are the salient points against this belief:

1. The initial impact was slight, therefore most likely he had minimal damage to his neck and none to his shoulder. A whiplash injury needs to be from a high-speed impact to cause chronic pain.

2. The pain should have been felt immediately after the accident, yet he actually felt pain two days later at work while his boss was giving him a dressing down.

3. The pain mainly comes on at work, where he is stressed. He has a difficult boss and since the pain started, his work has not really been up to scratch.

Sitting at home and using his laptop doesn't flare his pain in the same way.

4. The pain tends to improve if he walks and moves around. He can still ride a bike and jog without flaring his pain. If this was a significant whiplash, these activities should flare his pain. However, he has largely stopped because the pain has made him feel somewhat depressed. This suggests his neck is actually ok and the pain is coming from Reactive pain. Also the depressed feeling has added to his pain.

5. All treatments of his neck and shoulder – chiropractic, physiotherapy, osteopathy – help short term, but the pain returns. This suggests the underlying cause is not simply physical.

6. Lastly, mild wear and tear in the spine is such a common finding in a 55 year old especially, and most people with this don't have pain.

"Your honour, all of this evidence suggests the primary problem does *not* lie in his neck and shoulder, but is rather Reactive pain cued by triggers in his stressful work environment. He also has some associated early depression that further winds up his pain system and feeds the pain. He needs to address these factors to get better."

With this evidence in front of him, Tom's inner judge then speaks:

"It is clear to me that Tom has 'used' the minor accident to explain the pain. He has ignored the more important life events and stressors in favour of the safer, physical answers, which is why he is no better three years later.

"Therefore my judgement is:
1. Tom's primary problem lies in his pain system, not in his neck.
2. The pain came on whilst he was using the word processor at work and being yelled at by his boss. These are the main cues to turn on his pain amplifiers. The fact he can type at home and not have much pain is proof of this."

The court convenes, and Tom makes his decisions. My ongoing treatment plan is this:

1. I need to talk to my boss about the work situation, even if this is very difficult, because I now recognise this is an underlying driver of my pain. Having it all out in the open will give me the opportunity to find some solutions.

2. I'm going to start practicing the other keys including mind/body techniques [8,9,10] (see chapter 7), breathing [11,12,13] (see chapter 9), and posture (see chapter 13).

3. Every time I feel the pain at work, I'm going to remind myself that my neck is fine. The only reason I'm feeling pain is because of my Reactive pain pattern.

4. I'm going to start regular biking on the weekend and walking after work during the week. This is to improve my depression. If I'm still feeling depressed, I'll discuss this with my doctor.

5. I'm going to talk the whole situation over with my wife and best friend, because their support and understanding is vital.

6. Each week, I'll review how things are going and adjust course if needed."

Tom found the process of sorting out his Reactive pain exciting and fun, both intellectually and practically. He followed the system we had worked out together and after two months not only did his pain go, but his mood improved and he told me, "I have my life back."

Action Steps

1. Look for those times when your pain is triggered by a specific condition.
2. For each Reactive pattern, hold a court case in your mind (as described above) to see if your pain really makes sense.

5

Autonomic Pain

The third pain type is Autonomic. I know I'm talking to someone with this pain type when we have a consultation and they describe their symptoms. They come to the end, and I ask a simple but revealing question: "Is there anything else?"

At this point, they usually pause, and may even look a little embarrassed. Then, they give me a list of unusual and distressing symptoms – everything from hot and cold flushes, to dizziness, to irritable bowel syndrome.

In this chapter you'll understand how these seemingly unrelated symptoms can all be traced back to chronic pain. And in understanding this, you'll see how to eliminate them one by one.

To understand the Autonomic pain type you first need to understand how your nervous system functions. Your nervous system sends sensory data from your body to your brain. There are two parts to your nervous system – voluntary and autonomic.

The voluntary division is where you have control over what happens, i.e. I think 'move my arm' and my arm moves. This division includes all the things you do when you consciously move your body.

The autonomic [1] division, on the other hand, is only partially under your control. It cruises along mainly in self-guiding mode, doing incredibly important things like determining the rate your heart beats, controlling your blood pressure, your temperature, and running your bowels and bladder. All these functions are vital for life and they need to be constantly adjusted to match your environment.

Your autonomic nervous system has a sympathetic mode that winds things up, and parasympathetic mode that calms things down. The sympathetic mode produces adrenaline and noradrenaline [2]. This hypes everything up – heart rate, blood pressure, bowels and bladder.

The parasympathetic mode uses acetylcholine as a neurotransmitter and this calms everything in your system. You feel sleepy, relaxed – the same as you'd feel after a heavy meal.

Autonomic functions are not under your direct control, but they change to enable you to do the things you want to. For example, if I'm sitting quietly in a chair, my autonomic system will keep my heart beating slowly and my blood pressure low-level. My temperature will be appropriate to the room I'm in, and a myriad of other things will be automatically adjusted so I feel comfortable.

If I decide to get up, my heart will beat a little faster and my blood pressure will rise. And if the door bursts open and a very large and angry lion leaps into the room, my autonomic system will react without me thinking. My body will be filled with adrenaline and cortisol. My pupils will dilate, my pulse race, my blood pressure will shoot up, my whole body will be energised and I will leap off the chair and out through the window in one second flat... or be eaten.

These are completely appropriate reactions of my autonomic nervous system, and the angry lion response was a major activation of my fight or flight mode.

Now, take the scenario from chapter 2 where I smashed my poor thumb. Specifically, remember the point where the pain message reached the midbrain (or caveman brain), and it was interpreted as a message of danger. A switch was instantly flipped and I went into fight or flight mode [3,4].

This fight or flight mode is how we Homo sapiens survived a dangerous world. It's the same mode that saved our ancestors back in the savannah. And (if you're lucky), it's what saves you when you run into a hungry lion.

Your fight or flight response mode activates to help you escape a physical danger, and it does that very well. However, your autonomic system will respond in exactly the same way when you get a pain message. This is because pain usually means physical danger. However, if you are getting pain all the time from a malfunction in your pain system, this becomes a major problem.

It's a problem firstly because you cannot escape a message that arises inside you, especially if the message is a false one. I couldn't escape from the 'danger' of my smashed thumb. After all, my thumb is quite securely attached to me. But my fight or flight response kicked in regardless.

Fight or flight mode is costly to your body and mind. It's a mode that exists for a single purpose – to escape danger. Being in this mode – even a few times a day – will take a heavy toll on your body.

When you switch into fight or flight mode, your system is flooded with adrenaline and cortisol. These hormones are particularly unhelpful when you're in chronic pain because they hype up your pain system.

Hyping up your pain system will dial up your awareness of pain. The tension in your muscles will increase and your heart rate will speed up. Your breathing shifts into escape mode, and this turns on all the accessory muscles of respiration in your chest and neck. Fight or flight breathing further winds up your system (this is described in much more detail in chapter 9). Put these all together and you get a major increase in your pain and anxiety.

People in the Autonomic pain type have incredibly reactive autonomic systems. Their autonomic symptoms have become the main drivers of their suffering. The good news is there are simple yet profound changes you can make in your daily life to get back a sense of control and safety.

To understand the extent of the Autonomic pain type, let's look at the symptoms it can cause:

Temperature Variation
People in this pain type may feel cold or very hot (similar to menopausal women with hot flushes/flashes). The

temperature changes [5] they feel are not appropriate to the ambient temperature outside, and these hot or cold swings can be surprisingly distressing.

Heartbeat

With the Autonomic pain type you can get palpitations [5] – fast, forceful heartbeats. If you do have these, you first need to be checked by a cardiologist before ascribing this symptom to the Autonomic pain type.

Blood Pressure

Your blood pressure needs to be constantly adjusted depending on what you are doing[5]. However, with the Autonomic pain type you can get swings in blood pressure that don't match your body's needs. At times your blood pressure may drop. This will make you feel dizzy if you stand up or move quickly. At other times your blood pressure may be quite high (which is a risk factor for other cardiovascular problems).

Irritable Bowel Syndrome (IBS)

Autonomic dysfunction can cause irritable bowel syndrome [6]. IBS involves a malfunction of your bowel with cramping pains, loose bowel motions, and wind. IBS is quite common in people with chronic pain and it can make life very inconvenient and uncomfortable, as well as limiting social outings.

Irritable Bladder

People may also suffer from an irritable bladder [7]. This means you may suddenly have the urgent need to pass urine. You have to rush to the bathroom and sometimes people get caught short. This is both embarrassing and intrudes into social activities you would like to do but now feel uncertain about.

Hyperventilation

When your fight or flight response is turned on, your breathing becomes deeper and faster [3,4]. This is completely unconscious. Your breathing will automatically change from quiet, easy and effortless to more rapid and deeper.

Now as with all the other autonomic symptoms, this is completely appropriate when you are being chased by something. But when you are doing normal activities, over-breathing will make you feel extremely unwell and further wind up your pain and distress. (See chapter 9 for a fuller picture.)

*

These are the symptoms that may accompany the Autonomic pattern of chronic pain. All these changes are unpleasant and increase the stress you feel, which further increases the pain. A vicious cycle is created as pain and stress go around and around, feeding each other.

So how do you start to break this cycle? There are some rare people who can directly influence their autonomic system, but most of us can't. What you can do is change other key processes that are under your control. By doing this, you indirectly influence your autonomic system and shift out of fight or flight mode.

The easiest thing to start with is changing from stress breathing back to a normal, healthy, and appropriate pattern[8]. Fight or flight response activates stress breathing, but it's a two-way street. Changing your breathing is a powerful way to down-regulate a hyped-up autonomic system. When you switch to relaxed, diaphragmatic breathing it sends a message to your autonomic system saying 'relax, we're not in any danger'.

You're giving yourself time and space to calm down and return your whole system to normal function. There's a profound effect that sweeps your whole body when you breathe out. Your heart rate goes down, your muscles relax and your blood pressure drops. Once you're good at this, you can down-regulate your system in two to five breaths or ten to twenty seconds with diaphragmatic breathing.

It's a beautiful way to step back into control – both of your emotions and your physical body. Added to this, you're feeling a wonderful sense of calm and relaxation. You'll find out exactly how to do this in chapter 9.

Stress and Pain

Many people in chronic pain notice their pain intensifies when they're stressed [9]. So another way to improve their pain is to reduce the stress they feel. One way to do this is to interrupt habitual stressful thought-loops. This changes the chemicals your brain and body produce, which will then reduce your pain.

The problem with all this is that chronic pain is inherently a stressful condition. So how do you let go of stress when you're in pain?

Let's look at how stress happens. As your pain receptors are stimulated, a message arises in your nervous system. This message shoots up your spinal cord into your brain. Here's the important part: your brain will ascribe a certain meaning to the message. And this meaning will change completely how you (and your pain system) react.

Judith is a skinny middle-aged woman with whipcord muscles. She lives on her own and runs a small farmlet with a few cows, chicken and sheep. She has worked really hard over the years to be self-sufficient. She lifted a sick sheep onto a trailer about three years ago and felt her back 'go'. She saw a doctor after a few months who showed her the x-ray and mentioned in passing that her bones looked really thin (osteoporosis) and that her vertebrae were in danger of collapsing if she overstressed them with any lifting. This was devastating to her as it meant the end of her dream. She decided to keep going, but every time she heard a click or crack in her back, she imagined part of her spine imploding. She became increasingly stressed and depressed.

When I saw her a couple of years later, she was ready to give up. Her farmlet had fallen into disrepair. Her back pain had continued with big swings in intensity. But her main problems were constant fear and guilt that she was harming herself.

Sadly, the doctor had based his opinion on the x-ray alone, which is not accurate. I ordered a DEXA scan which showed that her bone density was only very slightly reduced and a repeat x-ray showed mild changes and no evidence of collapse. As we discussed this, her whole body relaxed. I encouraged her to carry on following her admirable dream. Her smile still sits clearly in my memory. When I saw her two weeks later, she was a new woman. Her movements were confident and her pain had reduced markedly.

Six weeks later, she showed me pictures of how she had cleaned her place up and told me that her pain seemed to have gone. She sent me ongoing pictures by email for the next couple of years and was doing really well.

Because Judith believed her back was being damaged from everyday use, she often perceived huge pain. She was constantly fearful, and this had switched on her fight or flight response, amplifying her pain. Her pulse rate was up, her blood pressure was up, her mouth was dry and her brain kept telling her she needed to escape from this very dangerous situation.

Her hyped-up autonomic system further increased her discomfort, her disability, her pain and finally her suffering. When her beliefs about her body changed, her fear went, and her autonomic system returned to normal, switching off her pain. In chapter 7 you'll discover a powerful practice to become aware of and change limiting beliefs.

Breathing and Stress Relief

In a previous life I worked as an emergency registrar in a busy general hospital. My beeper would go off and I knew there was another major crisis to attend. I would race to the Accident and Emergency department, and as I arrived there would be the usual disorganised frenzy of people rushing around attempting to resuscitate some poor person.

At this point, I trained myself to take two gentle, diaphragmatic breaths (as you'll learn to do in chapter 9). As I breathed out, I would pause and feel the gorgeous wave of relaxation whoosh down my body. While I did this, my head would clear and my body would feel relaxed and ready for anything.

I reckoned that if the person died while I was taking these two breaths, it was their fate. However, if they didn't then I would be in the optimum state to make the best decisions I could and help them recover.

This is an extreme example of what you can do day-by-day in your life. There are always times when life's pressures beat down upon you and you unconsciously turn on your fight or flight response (including stress breathing). At this point you have the choice to continue as you always have – letting your stress, pain, palpitations and anxiety spiral out of control. Or you can take two slow, diaphragmatic breaths, pause on the out-breath and focus on the beautiful relaxation that comes from this. What you've done here is interrupt the cascade that previously would have ruined your day. You have changed your state into one of relaxation, clarity, and control.

This is completely within your power, and you can use this practice in any situation. As with all mind-body techniques, the more you do this, the more potent it will become.

Catastrophizing

Another habit that induces stress is catastrophizing [10]. Catastrophizing is a formal medical term used to describe a negative-thinking loop. It involves leaping immediately to the worst possible outcome. It's stressful and bad for your pain system.

We'll explore this process in more detail later in the book, but for now one of the best ways to stop catastrophizing is to find out the facts about your injury. This is because when you've already had a serious and painful episode, your mind paints a worst-case scenario every time you feel pain. A fact-finding mission will help you stay calm when this happens, and a good place to start this fact finding is chapter 11.

Lastly, when it comes to managing an Autonomic pain type, an important concept is that of the cascade. For a lot of people, one thing – like a stressful day at work – can activate their pain. This is the first step of the cascade.

If you can recognise these processes – fight or flight, catastrophizing, hypervigilance – early on and stop them, then the cascade stops as well. However, if you don't recognise and stop these processes, stress and pain can build on each other. This starts a cascade of negative thoughts, emotions and autonomic changes which will then build your pain, create more stress... and everything spirals out of control.

When you recognise the early signs of a cascade, you can now take steps to halt it. Practices like breathing, questioning beliefs (chapter 7 and 9) and not catastrophizing (chapter 12) will keep you on an even keel, and prevent one small, stressful incident from turning into a day of stress and pain, and possibly causing a bigger flare.

As you get better at recognising these cycles and intervening early, you can extinguish them before they grow too big. When you make this a habit, your life will improve and an upward spiral will take you step-by-step into the realm of pain-free living.

Ruby slipped down the bank of a hill, twisted and injured her back a number of years ago. The pain never settled, despite seeing a number of eminent specialists. She had a recurring vision of losing the use of her lower legs and ending up in a wheelchair. Whenever this vision arose, a feeling of panic swept through her body. She felt embarrassed about this and so had not told any of her doctors. However, for some reason she felt safe to share this with me.

We explored where this could have come from. After about ten minutes she visibly started to sweat, became a bit weepy and, in a quavering voice, told this story.

When Ruby was a young child, she saw a man having an argument on the side of the road. He then whirled around and stepped onto the road, right into the path of a bus. He was struck and killed instantly. As a child, this experience sent a huge wave of shock through her body.

The fascinating thing was she had buried this experience. She never discussed it with anybody, but remembers having nightmares for a number of years. Life then moved on.

When she injured her back, what she didn't recognise was how her childhood experience now coloured any trauma in her life. It had set up in her an inexorable, catastrophizing logic. This logic stated: "Whenever things go slightly wrong, they will always get worse." Following this logic, when she twisted her back, it was inevitable that she would eventually lose the use of her legs. The panic that accompanied this destructive belief would create a huge surge of Autonomic malfunction that had been programmed at that fateful moment in her young life.

Realising this was a life-transforming moment for her. Once everything that had been hidden was laid out in front of her, she smiled and then really started to weep. Afterward she described how a huge fist that had been constricting her insides was released.

We then explored breathing, relaxation, and visualisation. Over time, as she made these techniques part of her daily life, her pain melted away.

Action Steps

1. Look for Autonomic symptoms. Recognise them and see how they connect with your pain.
2. Go on a fact-finding mission for your original diagnosis (chapter 11). The purpose of this fact-finding mission is to reduce stress associated with your future health.

6

Pictures on a Page

This chapter is all about beliefs. Beliefs are the unconscious bedrock of our reality. What we believe about our body and our health will determine what is possible and impossible. This is why we need a final examination of your beliefs before we enter the fascinating world of mind-body practices.

A historic example of the power of belief was athlete Roger Bannister. Prior to his record-breaking race, it was believed physically impossible to run a mile in under four minutes. Experts maintained that if you pushed your body that hard, your heart would burst. On the fateful day – May 6, 1954 – Roger Bannister proved it *was* possible. That same year, five others went on to run a sub-four-minute mile, and nowadays college kids regularly break four minutes.

What you believe about your body will determine what you can and can't do. If you believe there is something fundamentally broken or damaged in your body and it is unfixable, this belief will not only reinforce your pain, it may also make your pain unfixable as well. It is not until you embrace the possibility that your pain is fixable, that you will take steps on the journey to healing.

Whatever your diagnosis may be, I want you to know you are not alone. Hundreds of millions of people every year have chronic pain.

Here's how big a problem chronic pain is in the world today. In the USA alone, it cost upwards of $635 billion dollars [1]. That's billion with a 'b', and that's in one year.

All in all, it comes to more than the entire USA defense budget and costs more than heart disease, diabetes, and cancer combined [1]. Chronic pain is a growing health catastrophe, and one of the drivers of it is the beliefs emerging from imaging technology.

How do we form beliefs about our health and our body? Nowadays there is a particular process that has been enabled by imaging technology. This process occurs hundreds of thousands of times a year.

It looks like this...

You have reached a point in your journey through chronic pain where you absolutely have to have an answer and a solution. You finally get to see a medical specialist.

It is usually a very important person in a white coat who listens to your story, examines you and then sends you for investigations. These could be an x-ray, ultrasound, CT scan, MRI or other functional scans. You return to the specialist and now are in an incredibly receptive state of mind to hear exactly what the problem is.

The specialist will usually point out on the scan where the area of damage is and explain that this is where your pain is originating. It is there in black and white. You look at it and it makes complete sense to you.

The explanation, if it is well given, goes down to the bedrock of your beliefs. You internalise this knowledge and it sinks into the part of your mind where we all try to make sense of our world. It now forms the foundation for our understanding of what has gone wrong to cause this horrible pain. It then also determines your future.

Now this specialist is usually someone firmly entrenched in what's known as 'evidence-based medicine' [2,3]. This has been[1] the dominant form of medicine in the West for the last 30 years. And what evidence-based medicine values most is high-quality studies.

This means that to prove whether a treatment works or not, you need to trial it on large numbers of people, double blinded* to adjust for the placebo effect [4]. This then becomes one of the building blocks of evidence. The evidence is stratified [5] – from Level 5 (opinion of experts) up to Level 1 (meta-analysis of a number of high quality studies) .

There is an ocean of knowledge that guides the medical profession. This ocean is full of evidence, studies and data, as well as opinion. The person in a white coat giving you an explanation for your pain is dipping a ladle into this ocean of knowledge and then using that information to make your diagnosis.

---

[1] Double blinded means neither the patient nor the researcher knows which treatment is the real one, or a placebo. This takes out bias in the study.

So now I'm going to access that same ocean of knowledge and use its evidence base of research and studies to show you a totally different picture of what may be causing your pain.

Let's start by revisiting the day you were given your diagnosis.

Sitting there in the medical clinic, you hear the diagnosis, understand it and internalise it. It now takes up residence inside you as the reason for your pain, and the decider of what the future holds for you.

Except.

Except the diagnosis you are given is often based on entirely flawed data.

Dr Waddell was a visionary orthopaedic surgeon from Scotland who recognised that the normal medical model of scanning backs and then operating on them was not working. The study we're referencing is hugely instructive.13 In it we are looking down from 30,000 feet. It shows a huge increase in the incidence of pain in the general population dating from 1955 to 1995. This is measured as time off work and the data is adjusted for population size and therefore shows a real increase in chronic pain and disability.

So despite ongoing research, expensive new treatments, surgeries and medications, chronic pain is not getting better. It's getting worse.

In the mid-1980s the graph changes and becomes steeper and steeper. Something happened here to make the disability from chronic pain increase dramatically.

So what happened?

There are several factors. The pace of technology increased exponentially. Jobs became more uncertain, leading to more stress. People spent more time sitting down. As the pace of life increases, people find it harder to cope.

Another interesting phenomenon occurred. If I remember back to how I did medicine 30 years ago, and I compare that with what I'm doing now, my practice is far superior to what I used to do. However, the expectations of society, my colleagues and myself have risen even more at the same time. Therefore it is very easy to judge myself and to have others judge me as never quite good enough.

This doesn't only apply to me of course but to everyone. All of these factors add together to create a massive and growing stress as we all struggle to manage and survive.

Lastly, around the early 1980s was the time when MRIs and CT scans became widely available. Initially, this advance in imaging technology held out a seductive promise. At last experts could point at a picture of your joints or spine and say "There! That's what's causing your pain."

Everyone expected that now we could see exactly what was mechanically going on in the body, we could then fix it and no one would need to suffer from pain any more.

This would have been fantastic except for one small problem. From the time imaging became widespread, the incidence of chronic pain took off. What this means is that surgery and other treatments doctors used to fix the damage the images showed, weren't working.

So now there was a conflict or cognitive dissonance between what is and what should be. This further increased inner stress and reduced people's ability to cope with the pain.

Having seen the damage on a scan, people became afraid to move. They had the expectation that the invasive treatment they were offered would fix the problem. Sometimes it did, but all too often it didn't and, at times, made it worse. This increased the disability people suffered.

The logical conclusion is that all this fancy technology does not tell us what we need to know. Just by looking at a scan, even trained experts cannot tell the true cause of the pain[8,9,10,11,12]. Unfortunately, the belief in imaging to diagnose pain has led to many problems.

I work half a day each week in a pain clinic in a public hospital. One morning I saw a middle-aged lady from Myanmar who did not understand English and had come to New Zealand as a refugee. She had lumbar spine pain. Three months earlier she had seen an orthopaedic surgeon who had taken x-rays.

He had explained to her, through an interpreter, that the discs were very narrow and that she had 'bone rubbing on bone'. However, through her interpreter, her understanding was that her spine was crumbling and collapsing.

The surgeon went on to say that he could not help her and referred her to the pain clinic.

When I saw her I asked her what she believed was wrong. She explained through a different interpreter that every time she stood she heard some creaking noises and she believed her bone was crumbling.

When this happened, she pictured the inside of her spine falling to bits. Because of this she had become completely incapacitated. She needed help to stand and walked very slowly with the aid of a walker. She could only take a few steps and then had to rest. Most of the time she was wheelchair-bound.

Because of the misunderstanding with the surgeon, a huge deterioration had occurred in her muscle tone, back pain, and quality of life. And this was based completely on her belief about what was happening in her body.

I spent a long time going over the pictures with her and the interpreter, and at some point she smiled for the first time. She looked at me and said, "So it's not breaking?"

I nodded and said, "It is just fine." It was quite amazing to see the change in the way she held herself following this illuminating bit of information.

After seeing me, she had an exercise program from a physiotherapist and some more input from a psychologist. When I saw her six weeks later, I could hardly recognise her. The walker and wheelchair were gone. The years had fallen from her and she was moving quite freely.

She was completely transformed and went on to do very well long term.

This is a graphic example of the power of belief – both for harm and for good.

Let's take another look at what practitioners see when they try to find the cause of pain just by scans. And while we do this I'm going to do something called 'reframing'.

Reframing [6] is very powerful. You can look at something and see it a certain way. Then you can put a different frame around it, and the meaning of it changes completely.

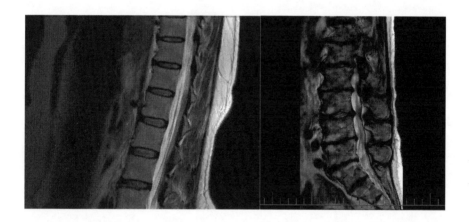

The MRI on the left is a pristine spine. You can see everything is smooth, the bones are spaced nicely, and the discs are large with fluid in the centre to help them act as 'shock absorbers'.

The picture on the right is very different. The bones are irregular. There are narrow disc spaces. The discs are dry and they bulge both forward and backward. On the whole, the picture is not nearly as pretty.

Medical science puts a frame around images like this. It says: 'This is a disease.' Spines like this are given negative labels like: degenerative disc disease, narrowing of disc space, osteophytes, impinging, damaged, stenosis and spondylosis. All these names convey the idea that this is a damaged spine. It's very easy to point to this as the cause of your pain. It's a logical thing to do.

Now this is where the reframing comes in.

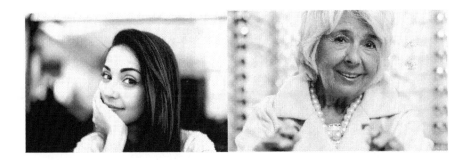

If we use the same criteria as the experts looking at your spine, the person on the left has normal skin and the person on the right has completely degenerated and dehydrated skin. The serious sounding medical term for this is actinic keratosis. With the previous logic, we could further diagnose that because this person's face and skin is so desiccated, they also probably have pain, low energy, a lack of joy, a depressed view of the future, and all the other things you might suppose someone would have with such terribly damaged skin.

I'm now putting another frame around the picture. The lady on the right has a beautiful face. A face that has been 'lived in'. Those aren't wrinkles, they are laughter lines. This lady has lived a full and rich life. She has wisdom and experience.

In short, she is someone you would love to be your grandmother.

Her wrinkled skin is not a disease like actinic dermatitis or terrible damage. It's just a natural change of a body ageing gracefully.

Here's the thing: the spine you saw is exactly the same. It probably belongs to a similar person. It's a spine that is lived in, that has been used and taken the knocks of life. It has adapted wisely and because of this, it works just fine. It doesn't look the same as a younger spine, but can be perfectly functional.

It would be lovely to say when you're born, you would live forever and nothing would change. But that's not the case. You can see this older spine as an evolution and adaptation to life.

Here is the natural process of how the one spine becomes the other spine. One day you've been twisting, working and lifting, and as you do this you make one extra movement and a small tear occurs in the wall of the disc. The disc is a strong structural element that sits between your vertebrae so that normally as you move around, the bones don't touch each other.

Now this tear weakens the wall of the disc and as you move, the edge of the upper vertebral body comes into contact with the lower one. Now there are two sharp edges touching each other and that can be uncomfortable.

Your body can't recreate the disc wall, because discs have a poor blood supply. But your bones have an amazing blood supply. So instead of trying to rebuild the disc, your body adapts the bone. It starts growing a ledge out. This ledge stabilises the segment and increases the surface area of the bone that comes into contact with the other vertebrae. This is like building a buttress to stabilise your vertebrae.

When you look at it under an x-ray, you can see this as a spiky growth. It's called an osteophyte and is given a negative connotation. But the truth is that it isn't a negative disease process. It's a clever adaptation of your body to strengthen and stabilise your spine. It only looks like a spike because you are seeing it from the side.

This process will continue until the segment is stabilised. Once the process finishes, the pain usually settles.

Pain from arthritis and joints actually decreases as people age [7]. This is because your bones are finishing their adaptive process. It's interesting; as you age, the scans of your spine and joints will continue to look worse. But despite this, over the general population, the amount of pain we feel decreases.

Once the process is finished, you will usually have less range of movement, but certainly enough to do normal activities. Your body will have stabilised the spinal segment or joint. In the spine, the vertebral ledges will sometimes grow even to the extent that they create a natural spinal fusion.

Your body does this fusion much better than a surgeon, however. Your body makes changes only where they are necessary. It keeps the part of the disc that is still useful, and grows bone where the disc isn't functioning.

Your body can change and adapt in the same way a tree does. It doesn't look as pretty (although perhaps it looks more beautiful to a discerning eye), but it is just as strong, healthy and able to function.

So with this new and empowering information, you can now understand why the majority of people with 'abnormal' scans and wear and tear in their joints actually have little or no pain.[10,11,12]

When ultrasound scans were first being developed, people were able to see the 'soft' tissues like ligaments and tendons. They started scanning painful joints. They did scans of people with shoulder pain and uncovered many instances of wear and tear. They could see frayed tendons and cartilage that was damaged. And if this was all they did, it would be easy to point to the damage and say, "that's why you have shoulder pain."

However, these same scientists did scans of the non-painful shoulder because they wanted to understand this new technology. And to their surprise they usually found just as much damage and wear and tear in the shoulder that didn't hurt [8,9].

In fact, at the highest level of evidence-based studies, medical scientists and statisticians have concluded that there is a very limited relationship between what can be seen on a scan of your back and whether you feel pain.[10,11,12] This includes x-ray, MRI and CT scans. All too often they do not show the true source of the pain.

To put it another way, you could take one hundred people with scans that showed similar damage to their backs, and some of them would have pain while others would have none. But their scans would look very similar.

I saw Gabrielle today (the day of writing this page). She was similar to many other patients I have seen. She had significant low back pain with sciatica. She saw a surgeon and her MRI showed prolapsed discs at the two lowest levels of the lumbar spine at L4/5 and L5/S1. The rest of her MRI was completely normal.

Because she was only in her 30s, the surgeon initially performed a small operation where he just trimmed back the damaged disc walls. When she woke from surgery, her pain was completely unchanged. She was understandably very disappointed.

She saw the surgeon again and he said now she would need to have the disc removed at both levels and have a spinal fusion operation. This is a much larger operation and involves taking bone from her pelvic rim and putting the bone in the space where the discs were. It also involves inserting screws and rods to hold the whole area in place.

She had significant pain following the surgery – this was to be expected. But as the weeks and months passed, the pain never went away. In fact the pain following the surgery was worse.

On review, the surgery was well done – the discs were removed and the bone grafts had taken. However her pain was unchanged.

How is this possible?

Because Gabrielle's – and so many other people's – pain was not coming from the damage shown in the MRI. It was amplified pain coming from her malfunctioning pain system.

This is how people can get a disc removed and still have pain in the same area. They can get two vertebrae fused and still feel the same pain.

So now, I invite you to review the explanation you have been given for your pain. And ask yourself: are you open to the possibility your pain is not being caused by physical damage but could be coming from your pain system?

Pull out your scans and images (if you have them) and reframe them. Look at them and say to yourself: "I may well be seeing changes from a naturally ageing and quite normal spine."

Finally, ask yourself this incredibly important question:

"Does the explanation I've accepted
for my pain <u>really</u> make sense?"

When you're able to set aside this explanation (at least for the time being), you are ready to embark upon the next important part of your journey. You are going to learn how to reset your pain system.

Before we start this next step however, I want to tell you about the forces arrayed against you, primarily those of self-sabotage.

We like to think we are one unified being, one personality with one goal and one way of doing the things we want to do. In reality, there are at least a few different personas within us, and not all of them want the same things.

This is another manifestation of the enemy within. Life can be viewed as a constant battle of good against evil, of growth against diminishing, of understanding against ignorance. We are all striving to be better, more compassionate and wiser beings. To grow, you need to be able to recognise the part of you that aims to bring you down and clip your wings in all its many forms.

Forewarned is forearmed, and the most common type of self-sabotage is refusing to accept the possibility that something you strongly believed is not true.

I remember a man I saw who had lived with pain in his thoracic and lumbar spine for many years. He was in his late-60s and had a CT scan showing widespread spondylosis (the changes of age, wear and tear). As with many people he had been given the explanation that his pain was due to these changes and it made perfect sense to him. However, all the many treatments he had tried had not changed his significant daily pain.

We talked and it became clear that his pain didn't really make sense in terms of a mechanical problem arising from damage in his spine. So I started to explain the possibility that his pain was not coming from his back, and that much of it was coming from a malfunction in his pain system. As I explained this, he crossed his arms in front of him, frowned and said to me, "So you think I'm making up this pain, you think it's all in my head!"

In part, he was correct – his pain was all in his head, but that is how we are all wired. We cannot 'feel' the pain in any part of our body – all pain can only be 'felt' and processed in the brain. However, all he took from my talk on amplified pain was that I thought the pain he had was 'not real'. Once this idea was in his mind, nothing I said would change this fixed point of view. He walked out of my consultation shaking his head and probably thinking, Yet another useless doctor.

This is a great example of self-sabotage and the enemy within. If this man had allowed himself to be open to another view on how his pain works, our conversation would have gone very differently. He would have been able to enter into the fascinating world of amplified pain – a world through which so many others have been able to return to their normal lives.

Instead, we didn't get to first base. Sadly this is quite common, and it's something we need to be aware of in ourselves. Not being open to a different worldview means our lives stagnate and we suffer unnecessarily. I know this from my own experience, and since then I've seen it in some patients.

It's hard because people in chronic pain are used to not being believed when they say how bad their pain is. It's important for you to know that when I talk about a malfunctioning pain system, I understand the pain is very real. The point is, it's not connected to physical damage. This means you can safely learn how to turn it down using the techniques in the next chapter, and get your life back.

THE
SECOND
KEY

7

How to Reset Your Pain System

Inside your head is the Cave of Consciousness where your awareness – The Observer – lives. Rapidly-changing messages from outside play on the cave walls. In your hands, you wield the torch of your attention. As the torch beam lights up one of the messages, it expands to fill the cave. It becomes your reality.

A pain message arrives with a flash, and the torch of your attention automatically moves to it. It fills your consciousness, and the message becomes pain.

Up till now, the torch of your attention has always turned to your pain messages and allowed them to take over your world. And therefore you live with chronic pain.

What you don't know, is that you have the power to direct the torch wherever you want. When you move the torch off the pain message and onto a different message, the amplified pain message shrinks, and over time it will diminish and disappear.

If you've tried 'ignoring' the pain before and it hasn't worked, it's because you still have the torch of your attention fixed on the pain message.

You have to learn how to MOVE this torch, and rediscover the power to turn it wherever you want. In this chapter, you will find out how to accomplish this.

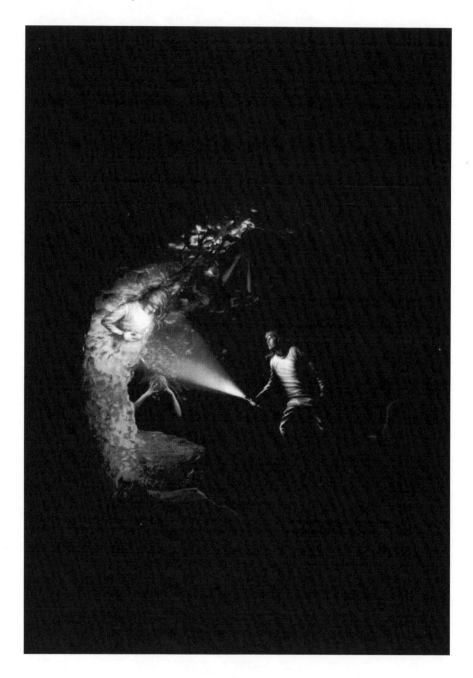

The second key to becoming pain free is to learn and then master one mind-body technique. When they first hear about these techniques, some people think that it all sounds too basic, and their pain is so intense they don't think it will work.

The battle to get your life back is won in small increments. Practice a technique each day, and over time you will notice – as I and many others have – your pain recedes. In fact it can literally melt away. I've seen this process take as little as two weeks, though for me it took twelve weeks. For others it's taken longer.

The First Key was to deeply understand the how and why of what you're doing. If you've read this far, you have that covered. This next key is to discover which mind-body technique works best for you, and then practice it constantly throughout your day with a curious and open mind.

When you accept that your pain is coming from an amplified pain message it completely changes what's possible for you and your pain system. This is because you no longer view the pain message as dangerous.

With this shift it's now time to start experimenting with mind-body techniques to turn down your pain. This isn't always easy. There's a reason I've spent the time explaining how your pain system causes your pain. Unless you've truly understood and bought into this model, unless you're willing to accept your pain may not equal physical damage, you won't have the conviction to practice a technique until it works for you.

It takes courage to challenge your pain. Getting to the place where you're ready to do this is a huge accomplishment. It took me seven years to get there (and some people never get there). However, by doing the groundwork and reading this far, you have arrived at the place where you can begin the work of resetting your pain system.

The techniques you are about to encounter are levers to permanently alter how your chronic pain behaves. When you think and feel in a different way in the face of pain, you are training your brain and your pain system to use a new pathway. You're re-opening the descending inhibitory pathway[1] that's lain dormant all this time. You're interrupting the pattern of emotion and pain [2,3] that has been amplifying pain messages.

There are many different mind-body techniques you can use to move the torch of your attention. After teaching them for many years I've found there is no one-size-fits-all. Some techniques will work well for some people, while other techniques will work better for others.

I had to experiment and find my own combination to switch off my lower back pain, and every time I teach a technique to someone in chronic pain, they end up adding their unique twist to make it work best for them.

So your task in this chapter is to get your first glimpse into another world. Once you have this glimpse, you need to be relentless in your pursuit of returning your pain system to its normal function.

Some people have great success with the simplest exercise – that of becoming the Observer. Other people find visualisation suits them better. Many people begin with one of the techniques described below and evolve them into a practice that's all their own.

The point is this: you need to experiment with these techniques until you find one that works for you, even if it only works a little bit at first. And once you've had this first glimmer that you could succeed, you need to double-down and practice this technique consistently as many times a day as you can.

Like all things worthwhile in life, these techniques are simple but not easy. Success will come with repetition until they become automatic.

I've put them in categories that relate to the three pain types. Some exercises will suit right-brained creative people. Others will suit people with a left-brain analytical bent.

In all cases, the important thing is to pick one technique and practice it diligently for at least four days. If you get some small success, double-down and make it your own; tweak it and twist it to fit you. If it doesn't have much impact on your pain then move to the next technique.

There is no magic pill except truly understanding what is going on, and then having the courage and determination to act on it. You discover which technique works best for you first by experimentation and then focus.

The rest of this chapter will describe techniques that have worked for many people to dial down their pain. The next chapter will go into how to master these techniques. Then we'll look at physical techniques that everyone – regardless of their pain type – will find useful. Finally, we'll look at some of the deeper issues that drive chronic pain, and what you can do about them.

Your Mind-Body Toolkit

Meet the Observer Within

This is the first critical element for learning mind-body techniques. It teaches how to go inside yourself and move the torch of your attention.

In any situation, there is you; but there is also the *you* that observes you. It's the part of you that is watching the goings-on in your mind and body. It is aware of, but separate from, your thoughts, feelings and ideas. You might call it the soul, self, original awareness, consciousness or *The Observer*.

This essential part of you observes your life from within the cave of your awareness. Normally, we are caught up in the constant whirlpool of our minds. You can feel angry, afraid, despairing. Most people feel like this when they're in chronic pain, and it's easy to be dragged down by these feelings and not be able to see a way out.

However, at any moment you can become *The Observer*. This is a choice you can make in a split second, and its effects are profound. When you become *The Observer*, you are separate from the workings of your mind. You are able to see what's happening. It is both powerful and freeing. In this state you are no longer at the mercy of your emotions or current situation.

Here's an exercise to practice separating and becoming *The Observer*.

As you sit reading this, mentally take a step back and assess the following: what is your emotional state? Your physical state? What thoughts are flowing through your mind?

A moment earlier, you were in the middle of these emotions, thoughts and sensations. They were dictating how you experienced the world. Now, as you catalogue them, you have become *The Observer*. You are one step removed from what you're feeling. You are simply observing the passing show. If you wished now to alter your state, you could introduce some new thoughts and feelings into your awareness. But with your new perspective, that may not even be necessary.

Practicing becoming *The Observer* gives you the mental space and clarity to do your other chosen mind-body techniques. It will also improve your life, giving insight into why you do the things you do, and make the decisions you make.

Next time you find yourself thinking or feeling in a way you don't want to, try this exercise. Take the position of being separate from the rest of you, and observe what happens next.

Techniques Best Suited to Hotline Pain

The Torch of Attention

Every moment of every day millions of messages are flooding into your brain from every part of your body. Unless you pay attention to them, most of them pass unnoticed. For example, it's unlikely you've paid any attention to your right earlobe while reading this. Or the little toe on your left foot.

If you turn your attention to your little toe right now however, you can start to get some information about it – whether it's hot, cold, comfortable etc. This information has always been supplied to you but until now you hadn't given it any attention so you weren't aware of it.

Your attention is the *torch* inside your mind. Whatever is in the torch light expands and fills your whole world. *Where the torchlight of your attention is aimed will determine your reality.*

Pain messages automatically jump into this light when they arrive in your brain. We are hard-wired for this to happen. This is fine if the pain message is caused by an injury, for instance if you've put your hand in a fire. You need this pain message to immediately grab your attention so you can prevent more injury.

However, if the message is being amplified by your pain system, it doesn't mean physical injury. Every time your torch beam highlights this message and gives it centre stage, you're making the amplification stronger.

Once you have the image in your mind of the torchlight of attention, it's time to use it in a different way. When a message comes to your brain that's part of your usual chronic pain, instead of letting it fill your awareness, turn the torch to another area.

Place all your awareness, in a mindful way, on the activity you're doing now. Pay minute and close attention to it. Let it fill your consciousness.

For example, if you're driving a car, look closely at the road in front of you; that's one sense – visual. Feel the steering wheel under your fingers – that engages your sense of touch. Listen closely to the car's engine – audio. Notice any smells in the air. And then, using all your senses, see how what you are observing changes second by second.

The feeling of warmth or cold... air on your face... sunshine on your back... light slanting through the window... see, hear, feel, smell – as if for the first time. This lures your attention outwards and away from the pain.

This is not the same as denying the pain is there, or trying to resist it or ignore it. Instead, you're changing the focus of your attention to your present environment.

Taking your attention off your pain and to your outside world is not easy to do at first. We're designed to give pain messages priority to keep our body safe. However, every time you practice turning your attention away from your familiar pain and onto something else, you will become better at it.

As you practice and master this technique, you will notice the amplified pain message coming up less often, and with less intensity. It takes dedication, and a firm belief that the message demanding your attention is, in fact, fake – a 'spam' pain message from your pain system. When you're firmly resolved this is the case, you'll be able to give spam-pain messages the attention they deserve – zero.

It's for this reason we've spent the time understanding the problem. Because it's likely in your search for a cure you've been given dozens of physical reasons for pain – from damaged discs to muscle imbalances. Against the myriad of physical explanations for your pain, you need to hold up this explanation, and over time you'll strengthen it with your experience of turning down your pain with just the power of your attention.

One superb variation of this technique is to place the torchlight of your attention on a part of your body that's comfortable. For example if you have a painful right shoulder, put your attention on the left shoulder.

Colour and Shape Visualisation

This technique is suited for people with creative and visual minds. Here's how it works:

Every time you feel your pain, you're going to alter the way you perceive it. To do this, give it a shape, colour, size and weight. This alters the way the pain message is received in your brain, and prevents the emotions it usually triggers.

Picture the pain as an object as vividly as you can. For example, a pain in your neck and shoulder could feel like a bright red sausage about six inches long and three inches wide. It could pulse and twist as you move.

Once you've created a strong picture of the pain as a physical entity, change it in some way. If it's red (painful), see a cool blue colour starting to permeate through it. If it's large and heavy, see it shrink in size and become lighter.

Once you've done this visualisation as concretely as you can, turn your attention back to whatever it is you were doing. Fill your awareness with your current task. After a few minutes, return your attention to the painful area and picture the pain once more. See its colour, shape, size and weight. Just be curious.

At this stage, most people will note a change in the visualisation. The pain has become smaller, it doesn't feel as intense, and it's less powerful.

Keep repeating this practice – altering how the pain looks and feels and turning your attention out into the world, then checking back to see how your pain has changed. Once people become familiar with this practice, many skip the first part and go straight to the soothing imagery. They flood the painful area with cool blue light, or send a soothing colour down the nerve synapses in the spine.

This technique works because it interrupts the typical pathways that amplify the pain message, pathways that have been reinforced over time. By giving the pain message a different meaning and processing it in a different way, you're building new neural pathways, and breaking the old connections between pain and emotion that keep chronic pain sustained.

Like all the techniques, the more you practice, the better you'll become. However, while you're practicing, it's important to let go of expectations. Simply observe the results of your practice like a curious scientist. This will stem the emotions of frustration, impatience and despair that block people from doing the visualisation successfully.

Nerve Message Visualisation

Quite a few people I've taught have adapted what they've learnt about the pain system to create a visualisation practice.

They picture the message coming from the place they feel pain, travelling along the nerve, and arriving at the junction with the spinal cord. This is the point where the message is either amplified or turned down.

Visualise the message entering the nerve junction and coming to a cool, soothing place. See the message diminish in size and become just a normal message – conveying a sensation of ease and comfort.

Here's a variation on this visualisation that worked for one lady:

Andrea loved the idea that there was a spam message carried by a tiny man running along her nerve. She could visualise this very clearly. As he reached the nerve junction in her spinal cord, she would 'swipe' her mental finger across the message as though it were a notification on her smartphone. The pain message would just disappear. This was her creation and it worked stunningly for her. The pain that had previously dominated her life rapidly became less intrusive and over several months, it disappeared.

Techniques for Reactive Pain

Recognition and Questioning

When you recognise your pain doesn't make logical sense, Reactive pain patterns start to lose their power. To accelerate this process, you need to become like a skilled prosecutor in a court of law and interrogate your pain. Use your logic to question whether your pain is totally consistent in how it behaves. When you find an inconsistency, it is proof your pain is not being caused by physical damage.

For example, *Richard had pain whenever he sat in a car for more than thirty minutes. But, he could fly across America with no pain.* This is a classic example of a Reactive pain. There is no medical reason why one would hurt and the other wouldn't. Until now he had a physical explanation for the car seat pain. He had to abandon that in the face of this evidence, and started using mind-body techniques to disrupt this pain.

Here are some more real-life examples of interrogating your pain:

'If I can be pain free when I'm busy, why does my pain come up when I relax?'

'If I can have less pain while on holiday, why does my pain return when I'm back in my normal routine?'

'If my pain is worse in the afternoon, why isn't it bad in the morning?' (or vice versa)

'If my pain is worse at home, why is it better at work?' (or vice versa)
'Why does it hurt when I walk on the pavement, but I'm fine to go hiking in the hills?' (or vice versa)

You're asking the question: "If my pain is absent at one time, or for one activity, then why does it appear at other times when the mechanical stresses are virtually the same?"

In essence you're asking: "Does my pain REALLY make sense?"

For many people I've seen over the years, logically questioning Reactive pain has been the catalyst to turn down their pain system. Once you realise without a doubt your pain is not coming from physical damage, you can stop the feelings of anxiety that come with it.

I've seen people go from thinking, *my back is about to break in half!* to *this is a nonsense pain message and I'm going to give it the attention it deserves - zero!*

The first thought means your pain will take over your whole consciousness and you'll feel much more pain. The second thought means the pain will be less, and be there for a shorter time. When people repeat the second thought until it becomes habitual, they reset their pain system, and over time their pain goes away.

Once you've used your logic to uncover your Reactive patterns, setting new expectations is the next powerful tool to reprogram your pain system. For example, if your pain wakes you at night, then before you go to bed take a few minutes to explain to your pain system that from now on everything is going to be different. You know what it's up to, but tonight your sleep will be deep, restorative and unbroken. You will wake just before your alarm goes, refreshed and ready for the new day.

This may seem like too simplistic a way to approach the problem, except for one point – it works for a lot of people. Firmly telling your pain system to stop sending you spam messages at night is often enough to break this pattern, because you then activate your descending inhibitory pathways. After all, it's been faithfully following a completely unhelpful program all this time, so why not give it a new and beneficial program to follow?

The key part is understanding. Once you understand your pain is not dangerous, that it's just an amplified message, then this 'talking to your pain system' has real power behind it. Your emotions of fear and anxiety are no longer reinforcing your pain. Over time the pain becomes less and less intrusive, and gradually disappears.

For some people recognition alone is enough. Others find they need to also take one of the Hotline techniques, practice it, and apply it whenever their Reactive pain appears.

Murray was a 45-year-old travelling salesman who originally injured his back four years ago. He slipped down a wet embankment and landed awkwardly on his butt. He had awful pain in his lower back and buttock whenever he drove his car, and especially getting out of it. However, he was able to sit in other chairs with minimal pain, and was fit enough to play a game of tennis.

His breakthrough came when he put together the picture of his pain patterns and saw it didn't make sense. The next day, he drove his car, and when it came to get out of the car – something that usually caused him agony – the thought arose: There's nothing wrong with my back – it only hurts!

He found this thought very empowering, and leapt out of the car seat with just a minor twinge of pain. Following this, the pain problem lost its sting, and these days, he's pain free.

Techniques Best Suited for Autonomic Pain

The Treasure Hunt.

Autonomic pain is strongly linked to emotions and stress. As an emotion sweeps across your mind, you have an immediate autonomic response to it, which then creates a whole negative downward spiral into pain.

To break this cycle, we need to get to the bottom of it. Emotions are the result of negative thoughts. We have all created or even cultivated certain recurring negative thought-loops which are linked to our pain. These have their beginnings in our past and are then polished and grooved in our minds over time. Beneath these thought-loops lurk beliefs, and these are what we need to change in order to stop Autonomic pain.

So let's see this as a treasure hunt. The treasure you're seeking to uncover is the belief under the thoughts and emotions. Because they are often well hidden, you may struggle to find these beliefs.

Therefore, as with all treasure hunts, there are clues to follow. The first clue to uncovering your beliefs is your emotions.

Emotions do not exist in a vacuum. What drives each emotion will be a specific sequence of thoughts stuck in a loop. Feelings of despair or frustration are the most common clues to follow.

When you see the emotion as a clue to uncover your beliefs, you can change your reaction to it. This can be profound. The next time you feel frustration, despair, sadness, fear or some other powerful negative emotion, instead decide: 'I will not go down the path I have trodden so many times before. I will now see it for what it is and instead I will go deeper.'

When you feel the pain and then the rush of emotion, the first task is to notice exactly what the emotion is. Give it a name in a sentence, for example, "I am now feeling sad/frustrated/disappointed/angry."

This takes you one step away from the emotion so you are able to look at it from the outside. The next stage is to be quiet for a few breaths, and notice exactly what thoughts are running through your mind.

For many people, an emotion like frustration will be accompanied by thoughts like, *I've tried everything and I still have the pain; will it ever end?* Or, *I'm never going to get better and will end up in a wheelchair; my body is broken and I need an operation to fix me; I will never amount to anything because this pain is ruining my life.*

When you become aware of these underlying thoughts, it changes the internal process that previously had a life of its own, and therefore had huge power over you. You are no longer the victim of these circling, destructive thoughts. Now you are merely observing them so you can follow the path deeper.

Like a good lawyer interrogating a suspect, you look at these thoughts and ask the powerful question: "Is this true or not?"

We all have within us a truth sense. You can use this to discern whether something is true, or just a creation of your mind. When you apply this truth sense to the negative thoughts, most of the time you will find they are not actually true. This realisation alone is often enough to change your emotional state.

Keep following the thoughts deeper and deeper and applying the same question: "Is this true or not?" At some point you will reach the foundation – the underlying belief.

Beliefs often have their roots in your past, sometimes as far back as your childhood. A belief such as 'I'm not good enough' can drive many negative thoughts and emotions. These beliefs took root in your childhood and then carried on for the rest of your life.

You may recognise the foundational belief as something you have walled off. You may suddenly remember the words somebody used or an experience you had carefully hidden away. This illumination indicates that you have found one of your fundamental beliefs.

Once you see the belief in its original place and time, and you observe how the whole thing occurred in the first place, you can bring your truth sense to bear. You can use your judgement and view it with adult eyes. Once you view it thus, the belief loses its power over you.

Martha had chronic pain for much of her life. When we looked into how she did things, we were able to determine a particular pattern of behaviour that was driving her chronic pain, (and that will look into in chapter 12).

The key was that Martha's mother also had chronic pain for much of her life, as had her grandmother. The experience of her mother constantly in pain and being unable to do many things had coloured her view on what her body was capable of, and what her future was likely to hold. She had unconsciously picked up emotional habits and patterns of behaviour from her mother and grandmother that sustained her chronic pain.

When she examined the habits and underlying beliefs about herself, she was able to start living a more normal, active life. After a time, her chronic pain shrank to just a minor part of her life. She returned to doing many of the things she had denied herself.

To uncover and change hidden beliefs, here are the **action steps** to do through the day:

1. When you feel a negative emotion, stop, and give it a name.
2. Grow quiet and listen to the thoughts accompanying the emotion.
3. Observe these thoughts and ask: "Are these really true?"
4. Look for the underlying belief. Ask yourself: "Why am I thinking this? What is the belief underneath this thought?"
5. Keep asking until you have gone through as many layers as you can.
6. Refocus your thoughts on what you actually want. Where do you want to be in six to twelve months? How do you want your health to be? With this in mind, create a new belief about yourself.
7. When you feel the emotion rising again, go through these steps and, at the end, substitute this new belief for the old.

When you create this new habit two things will happen. First, you'll be interrupting the loop you've been unconsciously playing where pain causes a negative emotion, which hypes up your autonomic system and causes more pain.

Secondly this practice will allow you to create new beliefs based on a more accurate view of reality, and based on where you really want to go in your life. Over time, these new beliefs will become your norm, and your Autonomic pain will dissipate.

I cannot overstate how important it is for you to do this in order to get out of pain. Belief governs what you perceive, and where your awareness and attention goes. Moment by moment, this creates your reality.

Be curious. Curiosity opens your mind and causes you to look at things from a fresh perspective.

Negative beliefs stop you from noticing things that could bring you out of chronic pain. For example, my negative beliefs about my back stopped me from asking an important question for seven years. The question was: "Why is it I never have pain when I'm at work even though I'm doing the same physical activities as at home?" In answering this question, I was able to change my beliefs, retrain my pain system and get out of pain.

Breathing

Whenever you feel stress arising, do the breathing practice at the end of chapter 9. This dials-down the fight or flight reaction in your body that hypes up pain. It also gives you a focus that's separate from that which is stressing you. Slow, calm, diaphragmatic breathing has been a powerful tool for many people I've worked with over the years. Over time it becomes an automatic habit and a practice for calming your body and mind, and regaining normal life.

Mary is a delightful lady in her 70s who had sneezed eight years before and felt a sharp, searing pain that spread over the left side of her chest wall. Because she had pain in her chest, she had seen various heart and lung specialists. She had had numerous investigations of these organs and had been reassured there was nothing wrong... except she still lived with daily, intense, intrusive episodes of the same searing pain, plus a constant background ache in that area.

When the pain came on, she felt short of breath, nervous, sweaty, heart racing and occasionally had bowel cramps.

We discussed what was actually happening in her pain system and how her autonomic system in fight or flight mode was creating all these other symptoms. Chest pain is an inherently scary condition, and Mary had an uncle who had died of a heart attack at a family gathering years ago. We agreed a sneeze could not possibly be still causing her pain eight years later.

After recognising when she was stress breathing, Mary learned the correct way of breathing. Breathing correctly not only turned her pain down, her other autonomic symptoms dramatically improved, and in time her pain went away.

Again, Autonomic types will also benefit from applying a Hotline technique when their stress-triggered pain turns on.

So these are the mind-body practices that have helped many people reset their pain system and get out of pain. When it comes to applying mind-body techniques, I've seen a few people turn a 10/10 pain instantly down to 0/10. However, most people don't experience such a dramatic change. What usually happens is you try a mind-body technique and there is a small improvement in your comfort. The pain reduces a little.

This is a huge signpost though! Your pain may have only reduced a little, but the fact remains – you did something with your mind, and you were able to change your pain.

If you feel like you need a physical practice to accompany the mind practice, read chapters 9 and 10 (breathing and trigger points) for examples of how people have combined these two physical techniques, and then add them to your mind-body practices.

The people who've succeeded with these techniques take this approach. With a curious and open-minded attitude, they experiment with an array of mind-body techniques. Once they find one that resonates, and they have that first glimmer of success, they put their head down and go for it.

They consistently apply their chosen technique each day, many times a day. And then one day, they notice their pain hasn't intruded on their life for several hours. Or maybe even all day. I love hearing people describe this realisation to me, but for now, I want to talk about some other pitfalls that trip people up.

One stumbling block is the frustration and impatience that can occur when a technique doesn't work immediately. Some people start practicing the techniques with a 'This had better work or else' mindset. Or with self-talk that goes like this: "What's wrong with me? Why isn't this working? This will never work!"

This completely blocks the kind of awareness you need to correctly apply the practice. Often it will take several days of practice to start seeing even a small result from the techniques you're about to learn. I liken it to learning a new language. At first you need to stop and think hard before saying even the simplest sentence. But over time, the language becomes second nature, so you just have the thought, then speak.

The same is true for these pain-reduction techniques. The initial period involves hard work, but once the mental patterns are laid down, the results come easily.

As you learn these techniques you need to be kind and patient with yourself. As any person who's been in chronic pain for years knows, your store of kindness and patience runs extremely low.

However, beating yourself up while you learn to retrain your pain system will only wind up your pain system, and slow you down. Instead, try to rediscover the source from which self-love and self-compassion flows. I believe this is a vital part of healing yourself, and will only speed your progress.

Another stumbling block I've come across is the grief people feel when the techniques start to work. Their mind plays a trick on them. Instead of focusing on the present day, and the bright future, they feel a huge sadness for the years they spent in pain when they didn't need to.

This is a natural response, and it's ok to grieve for a time. But then it's important to move on and keep consistently doing your techniques.

Which brings me to the last stumbling block – consistency. Some people start seeing an improvement, and they're getting to a good, comfortable place... so they stop. This is like orchestrating a jail-break, tunnelling under the prison walls and then deciding to pitch your tent in view of the main watch tower!

Once you see a reduction in your pain, keep going. Keep practicing your mind-body techniques until they become as natural as breathing. This, combined with the other methods we're going to cover, is how you get your life back.

In the next chapter, we're going to look at how to accelerate your progress using a little known function of your mind.

Action Steps

Choose one mind-body technique to start experimenting with. For the next seven days, practice the technique whenever you feel pain. Approach using the technique with curiosity to see what happens.

If you have a small win – a time when you used the technique and your pain reduced – then double-down on the technique. Practice it as often as you can throughout your day and refine it by observing what works best for you.

However, if after seven days of trying your chosen technique it hasn't reduced your pain, then select another technique that's very different in character to the first technique and start experimenting with that one.

Once you find the technique that works for you, carry on practicing it. Over time, you may refine it to make it work even better for you, until it is truly your own.

From the selection of techniques above, everyone I've worked with has been able to find one that suits them. I would be really fascinated to hear from you which techniques worked, and how you adapted them to suit. You could send an email to info@lifeafterpain.com or post on our Facebook page: www.facebook.com/Lifeafterpain

Initially, it takes concentration to make your chosen mind-body technique work. But in the next chapter, you're going to learn about little-known mode in your brain, which can put this on automatic.

8

How to Turn Down Your Pain on Autopilot

"We are what we repeatedly do." ~ Aristotle
"The unexamined life is not worth living." ~ Socrates

Let's recap where you've got to so far:

1. You understand how you can feel pain because of a malfunction in your pain system – an amplification of nerve messages – even when there's no damage taking place.
2. You know about the three chronic pain types – Reactive, Autonomic and Hotline. You have a good idea of which one is your dominant type.
3. You've learned how our bodies can heal and be pain free even when scans, x-rays and MRIs show past damage.
4. You have started to learn and refine one or more of the mind-body techniques to turn down your amplified pain and reset your pain system.

In the rest of this book we will explore how you're going to use this knowledge to custom design a vehicle for you to escape from chronic pain. In short, you will discover how to get your life back.

Now that you know about mind-body techniques, you need to learn *how* to use them in your life. To do this, we're going to look at a particular mode of function of your mind. We are now entering the fascinating world of habits.

Most people think their lives are the result of well-considered decision-making. However, the truth is that most of the time we live on automatic pilot. We are creatures of habit. The habits we have created form the fabric of our lives for better or for worse.

Therefore, learning how to create new habits is an incredibly valuable skill, and one you can use for many things as you move forward. It's also the mechanism you'll use to alter your pain system, and your life.

In essence, until now, your unconscious habits fed your pain. You are now going to use a powerful process to build new habits that switch off your pain.

The classic definition of a 'habit' is: "an acquired behaviour pattern regularly followed until it has become almost involuntary."

Habits are invisible programs you run in normal life, and you run thousands every day. For example, you don't think about how you brush your teeth or tie your shoelaces – you just do it a particular way, because it's a habit.

Here's the key fact about habits: once your brain switches into habit mode, it powers down.[1] It takes almost no energy for your brain to function in habit mode. This is how you can drive to work – doing a thousand complex things – and not even remember the journey. Your brain was functioning in hyper-efficient habit mode.

The useful side of this is it saves a lot of energy during a normal day – allowing you to use brain power for other activities. The dark side is that if your habits are harming you, you aren't even aware of what you're doing.

Habits are not just physical. We also have mental and emotional habits. And chronic pain habits are usually a powerful amalgam of all three – physical, mental and emotional.

Amplified pain is driven by habits that up until now have been invisible to you. To undo them, you first need to recognise them and see the damage they're causing in your life. It's only then you can create new habits to replace the old.

How do habits work? And how do you create new ones?

If you want to go deeper into this topic, I recommend the work of Charles Duhigg, to whom we owe a debt of gratitude. In summary, there are essentially three parts to a habit. The first part is the cue or trigger, the second part is the habitual action, and the third is the result.

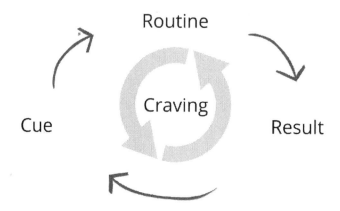

Let's use brushing your teeth as an example. The trigger or cue is the time of day, walking into your bathroom and seeing your toothbrush. The habitual action is the brushing of your teeth. And the result is you feel good because your teeth are smooth when you run your tongue over them.

We have myriads of these habit loops throughout the day. Some are positive – like tooth brushing. And others are destructive – like chronic pain habits. You need to know how habits work if you want to replace chronic pain habits with those that get you back to a pain-free life.

When you make your pain relief practices habitual it's actually easier to do them than to not do them. They simply become part of your day. You lay down train tracks and your thoughts and actions run on them.

There are two ways to create a habit. The easiest way is to join it onto an existing habit. It's like attaching a new train carriage onto the existing train – the track is already laid.

For example, every morning you do certain things, and they are usually the same things. Maybe you have a cup of tea, have breakfast, read the paper, and then brush your teeth. If you want to consolidate a new habit (like a morning stretch) you simply join it to one of these existing habits.

If you sit down and read the paper every morning while having a cup of tea, put a yoga mat there ready for you to complete your stretch. When you go to make tea in the morning, there is your mat, reminding you to stretch.

My wife used this to create the habit of doing kettlebell swings each morning. She knew that every morning she got up and made porridge for breakfast. So she simply had the kettlebell ready on the kitchen bench, and while the porridge was boiling she did her kettlebell swings. You can do the same for healthy habits you want to create. That's the first way to create a new habit.

The next way to form habits is by swapping old for new. This is important, because once you've spotted habits that keep you in pain, you'll want to eradicate them. It is very hard to stop a negative habit. It's like trying to unlearn something. (Have ever tried to forget how to ride a bike? Even if you haven't ridden for years, those pathways are still there, sleeping inside you.)

Eradicating habits is as difficult as unlearning a skill. So if you want to replace a chronic pain habit with a pain-free habit then you need to look at the cycle: cue → routine → result.

Instead of trying to stop the bad habit, you keep the same cue and you replace the negative routine in the middle of the habit loop with a positive one. This changes the end result. This strategy is how you integrate mind-body practice into your day.

Let's look at an example.

Jeannette had pain that was triggered by stress. In particular her boss stressed her out immediately – almost on sight. Just being around her at work would start Jeanette stress breathing and make her pain worse.

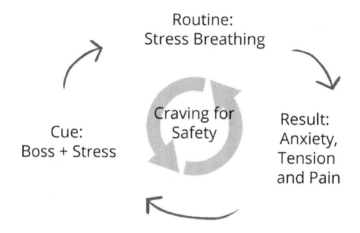

So Jeannette's boss became the cue for her to practice relaxed diaphragm breathing. Whenever Jeannette saw her boss, she would think 'breathe' and begin diaphragm breathing (which we'll be covering in a later chapter). Her boss now helped her to relax and breathe effectively, dialling down her pain. By the end, Jeannette would look forward to seeing her boss so she would remember to breathe calmly. This is a great example of how to take a previously negative cue and turn it into a positive habit.

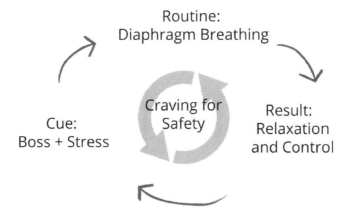

Routine:
Diaphragm Breathing

Cue:
Boss + Stress

Craving for
Safety

Result:
Relaxation
and Control

Take a minute now and think about the times during your day when you feel more pain. Are there any cues that prompt them? Are there any thoughts or feelings that continually arise, making you feel stressed, anxious, and in pain?

This is your chance to look closely at your life to uncover chronic pain habits. I'm going to go through a few common ones below; however, the most important work will be done by you over the next few days and weeks as you uncover *your* habits.

This reflection is a surprisingly powerful exercise. Becoming aware of and changing your invisible pain drivers takes you a long way on the journey out of pain.

Here are a few chronic pain habits to get you started in your investigation:

Searching for Pain

As we'll discuss in the chapter 13, searching for pain is one of the habits that will reinforce and keep feeding the pain cycle.

It's impossible to *not* scan your body. Instead, you need build the habit of searching for comfort.

Unnatural Movement

We're going to address this in more detail in chapter 13. What you need to know now is the habit of unnatural movement is a big part of Reactive pain.

For example: whenever I got ready to get out of bed in the morning the thought would arise – *this is really going to hurt.* This thought would trigger muscle tension and an abnormal movement pattern, which in turn amplified my pain. This pain-avoiding movement was part of the habit loop. I'd combined it with pain amplification every morning to unknowingly create agonising pain in my back and leg.

When I interrupted this habit loop, the thought *this is going to hurt* became the cue for me to relax, breathe deeply and move more naturally with the expectation that it was not going to hurt – or at least hurt only very briefly.

Within a few weeks of practicing this I was able to get out of bed normally again – pain free. Since then, I've helped many people regain pain-free movement for everyday actions like sitting, standing, and rolling over in bed.

We're going to cover natural movement in more detail later, but what you need to do at this moment is think and ask the question: When during my day to I anticipate pain?

Are there any movements that almost always cause pain? Write them down or remember them – we're going to explore altering them in a fundamental way shortly.

The next important part of unravelling chronic pain habits is examining your thoughts and feelings.

Thought and Emotional Pain Habits

It's really tough being in pain. When your pain turns on, this creates recurrent loops of negative thought and emotion. You're craving an answer and solution to your pain. You keep returning to it, trying to 'figure it out' and getting more depressed each time – very much like a stuck record.

Here are some common thoughts, feelings and beliefs that bubble up when people feel their pain:

- It'll never get better.
- Why me? What have I done to deserve this?
- The pain is going to get worse and worse.
- When I feel the pain, I know my body is breaking apart/crumbling/getting destroyed.

The thoughts and feelings that repeat in your mind every day are very powerful. They stem from your underlying beliefs about your pain, your body, and your future.

It's only when you become aware of the repetitive thoughts and feelings connected with your pain that you can start to change your underlying beliefs, and then your reality.

This may sound a little 'woo-woo' but consider this: what we believe about the world truly does shape our perception. And our perception controls what we can and can't do (or will and won't do).

Remember the refugee with the badly translated diagnosis? She believed her spine was crumbling away every time she moved. So she avoided movement as much as possible. All her paraspinal muscles stiffened – causing pain and disability – and her anxiety levels were sky high, further boosting her pain.

It was only after she seeded a new belief about her back (with my help and that of the translator) that she was able to make a full recovery.

New research into our brain's workings has shown that emotional and *chronic* physical pain light up the same areas of our brains.[2]

Imagine these two scenarios: a stabbing pain in your back that comes with the thought, my back is wrecked, *and* I'm never going to get better; and an emotion of despair and loss. Or the same stabbing pain that comes with the thought, it's just my pain system trying its old tricks. I'm going to move naturally and breathe; and an emotion of calm and determination.

The cue is the same – a sharp stabbing pain. The routine in the middle loop is the part you change from a negative thought and emotion, to an empowering belief, and a positive emotion. And, as so many people have found, you *will* get a different result.

Environment-Triggered Pain

Some of you have specific places that cue your pain. For instance, a morning walk or sitting in a car seat. So this is an environmental cue.

The way to change this habit loop is the same – use substitution. Instead of having the cue and then the pain, what you do is when you see the car seat or you go on your walk, this becomes the cue for you to practice your mind-body techniques.

You're reframing the cue. The cue will always be there, but now it has a different and positive meaning and result.

Katie noticed that her pain was worse in the morning. This puzzled her because mornings were when she tried to be calm and centred. She had a peaceful morning walk, and time for yoga and meditation. But this was when her pain flared. She had a busy life, and generally her pain lessened as the day went on.

This is a typical example of Reactive pain. It's dictated by the experience of the person, not the original cause of pain. I've met some people whose pain got better as the day went on and they were busy at work (like me). And I've met others who were better in the morning, and whose pain got worse throughout the day.

It's possible to justify either pattern with some creative explanation. However, when you look at the pain as a learned behaviour of your pain system then you can transform these patterns and get your life back.

So what did Katie do? She took the conditions of her pain-free afternoons and put them into her morning. In her case, distractions and busy-ness were her method of soothing pain. So instead of a walk with nothing to do but think about what hurt, she made her morning walk a time to talk with friends on the phone while attempting to corral a very active dog. Instead of stretching to calm music, she would turn on her favourite (dramatic) TV show.

By changing the routine, her morning became a busy, active time (like her afternoon), and she was able to create the habit of a pain free morning. Once she had ingrained this in her pain system it became the norm and her pain melted away.

Building Your Anchoring Habit and the First Hour of Your Day

An anchoring habit does just what it says on the packet – acts as an anchor to attach other habits to.

The best anchoring habit I've come across so far? Journaling.

Keeping a journal seems like a small, simple thing but it is actually huge. I encourage you all to start keeping a daily journal as your anchor habit. This journal writing practice doesn't need to be a complicated thing. In fact it shouldn't be. All you do is this: at a specific time each morning, take pen and paper and write down whatever is on your mind.

Don't make this a to-do list for your busy day. It's purely you writing down 'This is what I'm thinking and feeling right now'.

Once you've done that, write down the mind-body technique you're going to focus on today.

This anchor habit has three important benefits:

1. You get to externalise what you are thinking and feeling. Placing it outside yourself gives clarity and perspective.
2. Journaling becomes a daily reminder of your commitment to build new habits and get your life back.
3. It's a space where you regroup and track progress.

Some people find when they journal this can amplify their pain, as they're paying more attention to it and how they feel when they have it. It's a delicate balance. You're journaling to look for thought or behaviour patterns that trigger your pain. Take a clue from the word itself and be journalistic. The point is not to dive deep into and be dragged down by pain and emotions but to observe them.

Some people journal just for a week or two – long enough to uncover their pain-reinforcing habits. Others find they enjoy the journaling process, and continue with it. It's up to you how long you journal for, however it's a very useful initial practice.

The other tool to help you build new habits is to put visual cues around your house. Again these become reminders for you to do your mind-body practice.

Right now, under the radar, there are memories laid down in your usual environment that are triggering unhelpful things like Reactive pain, stress and anxiety. So what you are going to do is to lay a different foundation.

You are going to create new cues, and these are going to turn on new behaviours. You'll then insert them into your day, building new habits of feeling relaxed, pain-free and comfortable in your body.

As you reinforce these cues you will start to create new pathways in your brain. Your descending inhibitory pathway (the pain soother) becomes strengthened because you'll be activating it many times a day.

Pain Relief on Automatic

We've looked at the habit loop, and how you can change negative habits into positive ones. How then do you permanently lock these new loops into the uber-efficient habit mode? How do you now make them automatic so it's easier to do them than not?

The answer is: you need to repeat them many, many times throughout your day, and with your full attention. At some point, your habit mode will click in and they become automatic. From then on, you'll be on the winning side of the habit loop, and your life will be forever changed.

You'll be surprised one day to look back and notice your pain is much less. Almost without realising it, you have been through several hours – or even a whole day – without your pain intruding on your thoughts. We often get people writing in telling us this, and it's the '5-mile' sign on your journey home to comfort.

This is where you are going. It is the future you are headed towards, and this chapter will help you lay the foundation for it.

Action Items:

1. Start doing a journal every day. This becomes your anchor habit from which you will build the other habits.
2. To create this anchor habit, choose something you already do every day (like reading the morning paper) and attach the journaling habit to it. Journal either before or after this existing habit.
3. Write down any times you habitually feel pain, and negative emotions, thoughts or stress. You're looking for cues that set off your pain. Then, decide what positive thought and emotion you're going to insert into this habit loop. Practice inserting this new routine in the habit loop every time it arises.
4. Choose just one habit loop to start with, and continue practicing it until it becomes automatic. Only then move on to the next habit loop.

Next, we're going to look at one of the most simple and profound habits you can introduce into your life. With this one basic habit, you introduce instant relaxation, control and comfort into your day.

THE THIRD KEY

9

The Healing Power
of Breath

The third key to conquering chronic pain is breathing. You cannot get more fundamental than breathing. Because it is such a basic function, breathing often slips under the radar – we're totally unaware of its importance.

Most people think, *I breathe; that's good enough.*

The truth of the matter is that like everything else in life, you can breathe well, and you can breathe poorly. If you breathe well, you feel energetic, clear-headed, calm, relaxed, and in the control of your life. If your breathing is poor, or inappropriate to the situation, then there's a whole range of symptoms you may feel[1]:

- anxiety
- chest pains
- increased pain in general
- tiredness/fatigue
- tension in your body, especially in/across your chest
- visual disturbances
- dizziness
- hotness – especially your face
- inability to concentrate

- tingling in your fingers
- continually sighing and yawning
- a horrible feeling of air hunger/breathlessness
- tight jaw and throat
- headaches
- clammy, cold hands and feet
- erratic and fast heartbeat
- irritable bowel and bladder
- poor sleep with vivid dreams/nightmares

All of these symptoms can be scary. If you experience even one of them you can feel very unwell. You may book an appointment with a specialist, and have extensive tests done. Usually at the end of all this you'll be told: "Look, your tests all came back clear – you're fine." But you know you are not fine; you feel absolutely terrible.

Over the years I've seen many people who've had a long search to solve their pain and other physical problems. I've looked at how they breathe and told them: "Your breathing is completely dysfunctional, actually your breathing sucks!"

They look at me in total disbelief, but after they do the exercise we're about to do, their lives are transformed. Dysfunctional breathing is a wonderful diagnosis because once you recognise it (truly, knowledge is power), you can then change your breathing. This gives you a powerful tool to regain control in any situation, especially when you're in pain.[2]

Once you change your breathing back to healthy mode, you can change many other things in your life. Breathing becomes the key to unlock relaxation, awareness, and pain relief.

To get started, let's look at how breathing works.

Here's an amazing fact: your brain uses 20% of the energy in your body. This is boggling when you think of all the other structures you need to supply – your heart pumping blood, your muscles using huge amounts of energy as you move, your digestive system, and so on. All of those other functions are only taking 80% and your brain is taking 20%. It is a part of you that's very greedy, demanding, and picky.

As you breathe in, you put oxygen into your bloodstream.[3] Oxygen is an essential part of the energy pathways in every cell of your body. This is called the Krebs cycle. I learnt it in my second year at med school, and all medical students are tormented by this incredibly complex cycle.

In the Krebs cycle, glucose and oxygen come in at the one end. At the other end there is a high-energy bond created in a substance called ATP. ATP takes energy and distributes it around your body where it can then be utilised.

This process goes on in every cell. However, most of the cells in your body are not as picky as your brain. Your brain requires you to supply a specific amount of oxygen and glucose all the time. As you breathe in you pull in oxygen. As you breathe out you expel the waste product of the Krebs cycle process: carbon dioxide.

Now for the important part. If the pace of your breathing is appropriate to the needs of your body, you will inhale just the right amount of oxygen and you will breathe out the right amount of carbon dioxide. Everything is balanced beautifully.

If, however, you over-breathe – when your breathing is deeper and faster than the needs of your body – then all manner of problems occur. This over-breathing is called hyperventilation.

The needs of your body are determined by what you do. If you are asleep, your breathing will be very light, even, and slow. If you are sitting, it quickens. If you get up and walk, it speeds up again. Finally, if you are being chased by an angry lion it will be extremely deep and fast.

The needs of your body change all the time, however the needs of your brain stay the same. When you hyperventilate, your oxygen supply stays the same, but the carbon dioxide level drops, because you're breathing off excess carbon dioxide.

Now, carbon dioxide may be a waste-product of your energy cycle, but it still has a number of vital functions. It determines the acid-base balance in your body. If you change your acid-base balance, it affects the fundamental energy processes in every cell of your body. This in turn reduces the blood flow into your brain, other organs, and muscles.

Side note: this effect is used in intensive care units in hospitals when someone has had a severe head injury which causes brain swelling. Your skull cannot expand, so any swelling inside your brain will cause increased pressure and damage the brain as it presses against the skull. To prevent this, people in danger of brain swelling are then purposely hyperventilated – sometimes for a week – to reduce the blood flow into their brain and reduce swelling. That's how powerful this effect is.

When the acid/base balance changes, one other effect is a shift in calcium levels in the blood. This causes increased sensitivity in nerves and muscles, setting off pain and muscle spasm.

Hyperventilation gets worse when you are stressed. It is part of a huge autonomic change known as the fight or flight response (which we discussed in detail in chapter 5). The bottom line is, over-breathing will make you feel incredibly unwell, anxious, and stressed. It causes fundamental changes in your body that turn up your pain, and keep you trapped in the chronic pain cycle.

Even if you don't think you over-breathe, if you find yourself feeling stressed throughout the day, it's highly likely you're hyperventilating without knowing it. Changing your breathing is a powerful tool to regain control of your life. I've seen people resume their normal lives free from pain just by integrating the techniques we're going to go through now.

*

The series of exercises[4] we're going to do is what I do in my clinic when I see someone who is obviously breathing poorly.

When this happens, I explain what's going on and we schedule a special session just to get their breathing right.

I love these sessions because I sit quietly with the person, and as I talk them through the whole process, I mirror their breathing. By the end of the session we're both breathing together in a totally relaxed and cruisy fashion.

Fair warning, the first exercise is not going to be very nice. This is because to fully understand what hyperventilation feels like, you're going to have to experience an extreme version of it.

This way you'll be able to recognise in the future when you're hyperventilating. For this exercise it's important for you to be sitting down in a comfortable chair or sofa that has arms. It's not going to be a pleasant experience, but you can stop at any time.

Step I: Experiencing Hyperventilation

Take ten to twenty very deep breaths one after another. Breathe in as deep as you can, then breathe out as much as you can, and don't take a break between breaths – breathe as though you are running fast.

It's variable as to when you start to feel the effects of hyperventilation. At some stage, you'll probably start to feel uncomfortable, a bit dizzy and panicky – like you don't have enough air, even though you're breathing very vigorously. Stop doing the deep breaths as soon as it becomes too uncomfortable.

You will often feel heat in your face and notice tingling either around your lips or in your hands. Overall, you will feel just terrible. This is the classic effect of hyperventilation or over-breathing.

Now you know how hyperventilation feels. If you are hyperventilating throughout the day, it most likely won't be as extreme as what you're feeling now. But the effects are very real, and can be very distressing.

Step II: Understand How Your Breathing Works[3]

I have a question for you. It's very basic.

What organ do you breathe into and how big is it?

I ask this because over the years I've had many different answers, and it's important you know this so you can do the following exercise correctly. The answer is that you breathe into your lungs, and as you see in this picture, they are two huge balloon-like structures that live in your chest. They fill your chest and your heart is tucked in between them.

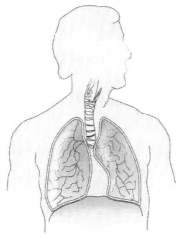

The chest wall that protects your lungs is quite elastic. There are muscles between each rib and the whole structure can expand and move as needed.

Step III: Exploring Your Breathing

I'd like you to lie down now and put one hand on your chest and one hand on your belly. Breathe normally and as you breathe we're going to do a lesson in awareness. Awareness is the key to breathing well.

As you breathe in, which hand moves more? The hand on your belly? Or, the hand on your chest? And as you breathe out, again, which hand moves more? The hand on your chest? Or belly?

Is only one hand moving? Or, do they both move?

Breathe some more, and use these questions to refine your perception of what happens when you breathe. In this exercise most people find one hand moves much more than the other, but both hands will move a bit.

Next, ask yourself: as you breathe in and out, which hand moves first – your chest or your belly?

There are many variations. You may find your belly kicks in first, or your chest moves first. Sometimes one of them will move much more than the other, then as you breathe out the pattern changes.

Which feels better? A belly breath or a chest breath?

For the next sixty seconds just be aware of the pattern of breathing in your body.

*

Answer me this: when you breathe in, you fill your lungs, and this will cause your chest to expand – a chest breath. So how can you have a belly breath?

The answer is that you use a wonderful structure in your body called your diaphragm. The diaphragm is a huge muscle dividing your body in half. It is shaped like a dome and sits at the base of your lungs. It attaches to your ribs and the front of your spine in two long extensions of the muscle.

As the diaphragm contracts it goes from dome shaped to flattened. As it flattens it greatly increases the volume of your lungs. In the picture below you can see as your diaphragm pushes down, it expands into your abdomen.

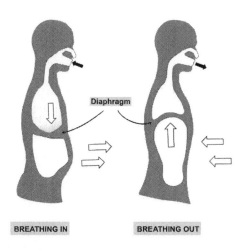

BREATHING IN   BREATHING OUT

As you breathe in, the diaphragm comes down and your tummy will expand outwards. And as you breathe out, your belly will contract inwards. This is what happens when you use your diaphragm to breathe.

For those of you with young children or grandchildren (like me) close your eyes and picture this child. What moves when they're breathing in? The answer for any child from newborn to three years of age is that their belly expands as they breathe in. Our most efficient mode of breathing is a belly breath.

We're all designed to breathe with our diaphragm. Your diaphragm moves lots of air, is very efficient and it's relaxing to breathe with. It is full of Type 1 muscle fibres, which are grunty and slow metabolising. They will work day in and out and never complain.

If this is how we're designed, then why do we have an alternate chest breathing mode? The answer is that this is our 'escape-from-danger' breathing mode.

Imagine you were walking along and came around a corner and saw a big angry lion. In this instance, you wouldn't breathe nice and slowly into your belly. You wouldn't breathe through your nose (which is part of the efficient breathing system we normally use). You would take in a huge breath through your mouth, turn and run as fast as you could, using everything you've got to escape. Instead of breathing into your belly, you would expand your chest as you breathed in. Chest breathing is part of your fight or flight response. It gives you an extra 15-20% so you can escape from danger.

Your ancestors did that and survived – that's why you're here today.

The interesting thing about the fight or flight response is that it isn't under your conscious control. If you remember back to the first talk on how our pain system works, the fight or flight response is controlled by the caveman brain – the primal part of us that's concerned mainly with survival.

Turning on your fight or flight response turns on chest breathing. However, this process works both ways. Chest breathing will kick you into fight or flight mode.

Nowadays we are less likely to be chased by angry lions. Instead, we may sit, apparently docile at a desk, tapping away on a computer while inside us, all manner of stress hormones are churning through our system.

In this situation, you're stressed, and therefore unconsciously you are chest breathing. However, *your body is not running as fast as it can away from danger.* This means you're breathing off excess carbon dioxide. This changes the acid-balance in your body, and you feel awful.

There's one other reason people use their chest rather than their diaphragm for breathing. It's for appearances sake. Perhaps when you were young you were told: "stand up straight and pull your tummy in – that's good posture." Many people also walk around with their tummy sucked in so they look trim. Both behaviours completely disrupt your ability to breathe with your diaphragm. It's like turning off your Rolls Royce engine and using a beaten up old Ford with flat tires.

Remember Step I – experiencing hyperventilation? Usually over-breathing isn't this extreme (except for people having a panic attack). What most people do instead is drift in and out of mild hyperventilation throughout the day. As stress comes on, they shift into using their chest more. As their breathing gets deeper and faster they feel unwell and out of control.

It's an unconscious attempt to escape from danger. The problem is, if you have chronic pain, the danger lives inside you and you can't escape. Your caveman brain doesn't get this, and so turns on hyperventilation. This causes the feeling of air-hunger and the carbon dioxide imbalance which further winds up your pain.

Step IV: Turning on Your Diaphragm Breathing[4,5]

This next part is where it gets fun. As you're lying down, breathe deeply into your belly with your shoulders relaxed. As you breathe in, feel like you are bypassing your chest. Imagine there's a tube running from your nose straight down to your belly. As you breathe in, feel your belly expanding, and as you breathe out, feel it dropping. If you find this difficult, then put a medium-sized book on your tummy and as you breathe in, lift the book up with your belly.

The usual rate of breathing in relaxed mode is about twelve to fifteen breaths per minute. It's a beautiful thing, just allowing your breathing to happen.

Do this for two minutes.

Now I'm going to introduce one more concept for you.

Take a huge breath. Fill your chest, belly – everything. Feel the increase in tension throughout your body.

Now let that breath go. As you reach the end of your exhale, pause. Experience how your body feels.

As you breathe in, there's an increase in tension. Breathing in changes your autonomic system. Your blood pressure increases, your heart rate increases, your muscle tension increases. Everything hypes up. As you breathe in, your brain is saying, "We need this oxygen – grab it."

As you breathe out, the autonomic tide recedes. Your heart rate drops, your blood pressure goes down, your gut slows down – everything relaxes. It's incredible. Every time you breathe out, it's a gift. It's your relaxation time. But you can only gain value from this gift if you are aware of it.

As you breathe in, make it a nice gentle diaphragmatic breath into your belly. As you breathe out, feel the relaxation like a wave sweeping through your body. Pause at the end of each out-breath for a second or two. Become aware of this gorgeous relaxation. It's yours whenever you need it.

As you do more of these breaths, your relaxation will become more and more profound. Feel the difference as you enter this state. Contrast it with times you're stress-breathing. In the depths of relaxation, let your body know this is how you plan to breathe throughout your day.

I learnt these breathing techniques years ago at a yoga retreat. It blew my mind how quickly I could reach deep relaxation levels. I then trained myself to enter this state in just a few breaths. This was very useful when I worked as a doctor in an emergency hospital ward and needed to make tough decisions with a clear and focused mind.

Step V: Using Diaphragm Breathing in Your Day

When you feel you've mastered diaphragm breathing lying down, it's time to practice it in two new positions – sitting and standing.

Try this: feel the ease of diaphragmatic breathing while lying down. Then, sit up and note what happens. For almost everyone, breathing sitting up is harder. This is because there is increased pressure on your belly as you become vertical. Often people temporarily lose the knack of diaphragmatic breathing. This is an important skill to learn, as we experience most stress whilst sitting or standing. So I have found a way to retrain your diaphragm so you can breathe well in any posture.

Lie down again. Breathe in using your diaphragm. Now, as you breathe out actively push the air out using your abdominal muscles. This will completely empty your lungs and create a space for your diaphragm to expand into. Do this lying down until you are confident in how it works.

Then stand. Breathe in through your nose, and as you exhale push the air out with your belly muscles. Keep going until there is no more air in your lungs. Then LET GO of your belly and allow the air to rush in to fill your lungs. Repeat this a number of times. Then dial back on the amount you push until your breathing is gentle and effortless.

Most people find they need to really concentrate to do this. Just remember, you are actually relearning an old skill. Everyone used their diaphragm to breathe as children; we just forgot how to do it as adults. So, be gentle on yourself, but keep going. Practice every day, initially lying down, then standing and sitting. Practice when you have no stress, until you can do it without trying. Then become aware of your breathing whenever the heat is on. Now you have the tools to change your breathing pattern and everything will improve!

Jack is a high-powered executive in his mid-50s. He lives an intensely stressful life, often rushing from one important business meeting to another. A few years ago he noted the onset of nasty headaches that arose from the back of his head and ended somewhere behind his eyes. These were associated with a feeling of heat and pressure in his face plus an unusual dizziness where he seemed to lose his equilibrium. They came on often in meetings, and were significantly impairing his ability to function.

He saw a neurologist and had an MRI, which was thankfully normal. He had hypertension and his physician increased his medication and added a beta blocker (which can both reduce blood pressure and headaches). Unfortunately the episodes did not decrease. He saw me because he wondered whether the headaches were arising from his neck.

His neck had some tenderness, but then I asked him to hyperventilate in my office. After five breaths he clutched his head and said, "Oh my God, this is it!"

We explored together how breathing can profoundly change so many things in your body. He learnt how to use his diaphragm to breathe in any situation, and especially he learned how to focus on and enjoy the relaxation experience that occurs with every out-breath. He practised breathing in the same way he did everything else, which was at the highest level. His headaches rapidly disappeared.

He also found he felt better in other ways – some obvious and some subtle. He realised he drifted in and out of hyperventilation many times during the day. He had done everything in his life at great pace and intensity, now he discovered a 'cruise control' mode in which he was super-efficient, but calm.

When he saw me a few months later, he told me this knowledge and practice had literally transformed his life.

Step VI: Breathing and Talking

We all spend much of the day talking. Often when we have an idea, we take a big breath in through our mouth and then keep talking until we run out of breath. Then we gulp in another huge breath and keep going in this way until we have communicated the idea.

This makes our speech pressured and our breathing dysfunctional. It is easy to slip from this into a hyperventilation state. The listener feels your inner tension and this interferes with their ability to truly hear what you are saying. This was particularly important for Jack.

There is a second way of communicating. Here you take advantage of the small natural pauses that occur with relaxed communication. These pauses appear as commas, full-stops, and other punctuation marks in writing.

You start with a small breath in through your nose. Then you speak in a relaxed voice until you reach the first natural pause. Now you take another gentle diaphragmatic breath in through your nose and speak until the next pause.

You are now breathing in through your nose, which sets you up for healthy breathing. Your speech is measured, your voice is relaxed, and your listener is given space to hear and understand fully what you are saying. This is immeasurably helpful for both of you.

Step VII: Breathing While Working

Relaxation breathing while you're lying down is a beautiful thing to do at the start or end of your day. However, while you're at work or around the house, you'll usually be sitting, standing, or walking.

Once you know how diaphragmatic breathing feels, you need to start doing it as you go about your daily tasks. First practice breathing while sitting, and then standing. As you practice more, you'll find yourself naturally breathing healthily without being aware of it.

The key is remembering to breathe well. One tactic people have found helpful is to put post-it notes or coloured sticker dots around their house and workplace. Put them in key areas like your computer, the steering wheel of your car, and your bathroom mirror.

The notes don't need to say anything, they're simply a reminder to breathe, and as soon as you see them, you'll remember to fall into relaxed and steady diaphragmatic breathing.

We're about to dive into an area that's interested me for many years, and which has long been misunderstood by the medical profession. It's an exciting exploration, because many people here find they're able to get pain relief in as little as 90 seconds.

THE
FOURTH
KEY

10
Trigger Points

A lot of people find my site – www.LifeAfterPain.com – because they're looking for a way to turn off their trigger points. This knowledge is the Fourth Key to living pain free, and a powerful aid in your journey. If you have no idea what a trigger point is, we'll start with an explanation, and then move on to more advanced knowledge of how they fit into treating chronic pain.

Trigger points were certainly part of my back pain. In the seven years I had chronic pain I was continually getting active triggers. Almost all people with chronic pain have trigger points, and they can be a major contributor to their pain. The good news is you can treat them yourself very effectively.

For many people with muscle pain, treating triggers is a godsend. I've helped people end years of pain because we found the main trigger point and switched it off. However, for people with chronic pain, their most common complaint is:

"I treat my trigger points and get fast pain relief. But the triggers keep coming back."

Once you understand what causes trigger points and put this together with what you already know about amplified pain, you'll see why this happens, and know what to do about it.

Trigger points are a micro-spasm within your muscle.[1] The trigger point itself is painful to the touch, and if you were to look inside the trigger-point complex (as it's called) you'll find the fibres pulled tight in an area within your muscle.

What is even more interesting is that when the trigger is active (in spasm) it acts like the trigger of a gun. The trigger fires and causes pain, sometimes quite far away from where it is. Each trigger point has a specific pain pattern. These patterns were mapped out years ago by Drs Travell and Simons[1], and some of them are quite unusual. Check the online bonus section of the book at www.6KeysPainFree.com for an interactive tool showing the locations and pain patterns of all the common triggers in your body.

For example, a trigger point in your shoulder can send pain up into your neck, and a trigger in your neck can send pain into your head and behind your eyes. A trigger in your upper arm can create pain in your elbow, a trigger in your calf can cause pain in your foot, and lower back triggers can cause pain in your butt... and so on. Because they're sometimes nowhere near the site of the pain, triggers are often missed as the cause.

The reason for these pain patterns is the fascia. Fascia is marvellous stuff. It covers all the muscles of your body. Any movement you do requires a lot of individual muscles to work together, and fascia coordinates them so they dance in harmony. Fascia is also richly enervated, meaning it's full of nerve endings. These nerve endings are why you get the complex patterns of trigger-point pain. And this is the origin of the term myofascial* pain – the broader description for this type of pain.

Underneath the fascia are your muscles. This is where trigger points reside. The spasm of the trigger is usually small, and when it occurs[2] it pulls a band of muscle tissue tight from one end of the muscle to the other.

Trigger points can exist in two states: latent – meaning it's there, but not actively causing pain; and active – causing pain. Latent trigger points contribute to stiffness in muscles, so it's well worth treating them if you want to increase flexibility and feel younger. Active trigger points can cause significant pain. I have seen people who've resorted to surgery for their pain, only to find out later their pain was caused by triggers.

So what creates an active trigger point? A trigger point is a neuromuscular process[2]. This means it's formed by nerves and muscles acting together. The way they interact shines a light on why they're so common in people with chronic pain.

Inside your muscles are millions of tiny spring-shaped nerve spindles. They're constantly sending feedback as you move. These nerve spindles have two modes of function. The first mode sets the length and tension of your muscles. Millions of fine adjustments in muscle tension is how you move smoothly. Even simple activities, like sitting upright, require seamless coordination between dozens of muscles. Little

---

[2] *Myofascial describes the two structures in this type of pain - where myo means muscle and fascial refers to the fascia.

babies spend months learning how to do this, but once we've mastered it we do it without thinking.

The second mode of the spindles is protection mode. When a muscle is stretched too far – for instance when you trip and fall – your nerve spindle senses this. As a stretch comes on too strongly, it sends an urgent message to the muscle to contract and protect your joints from damage.

This message zips from the muscle spindle to the spinal cord then back to the muscle in a closed loop **(1)**. The muscle contracts automatically – faster than thought.

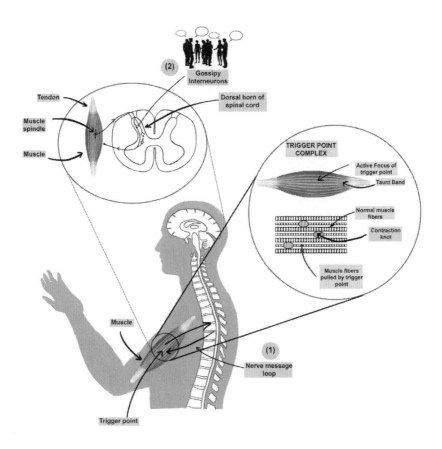

Active trigger points occur when this protective reflex switches on and doesn't switch off as it should. This neuromuscular malfunction can continue to cause pain for years if untreated. You need to interfere with this closed loop to switch the trigger point off.

So the trigger point is stuck in active mode, it's humming away in the background causing pain and stiffness. If the trigger point is the primary problem, when you treat it, the trigger melts away and the pain goes for good.

But what if the trigger point comes back? There are two reasons why this happens. The first is well known and easy to recognise, while the second is hidden and few people know about it.

In the first instance, the trigger points are secondary to an obviously damaged structure. If you have an injured disc, or a joint that's inflamed, it sends messages to the surrounding muscles to protect it. This creates trigger points. In this case, treating the triggers will only give short-term relief. You need to treat the underlying problem for long-term effectiveness.

What most health practitioners don't know is that a major cause of triggers returning is a pain system that's on hyper alert.

Let's look again at the area where the closed loop from a trigger point operates. It's the exact same area where Dodgy Don, Gossipy Gerty and the rest of the crew from chapter two hang out **(2)**. If your pain system is sensitised, they're on red alert. As a message from a normally-functioning muscle spindle comes into this area, it gets amplified by Gossipy Gerty and her interneuron friends. The message returns to the muscle, switching on the trigger-point spasm. This is how trigger points become part of the chronic pain cycle.

Here is the key point: *an amplified pain system sets off trigger points in the area of pain.*[3,4]

In this situation, only treating the trigger points is like trying to dry your floor without first fixing the leak in the roof that is dripping onto it.

This insight is exciting because now you have two ways of treating amplified pain. You can adopt a top-down approach using mind-body techniques to reset your pain system. And you can do a bottom-up approach: treating triggers to relax an area and prepare it for normal nerve messages. When you use these two approaches together, you get the best results.

Now you understand the connection between chronic pain and trigger points, let's look at the best way to turn them off.

The 90-Second Trigger Point Treatment

You're going to learn how to turn off a trigger point – effectively and with minimal discomfort. To do this, the most important thing is to be very gentle on your body.

It's tempting when you find the trigger point to dig in and try to kill it. This is counter-productive, especially for people with chronic pain, and can set off pain flares. What you want to do instead is gently sneak up on the trigger. I'm going to demonstrate how to do this on a very common trigger point.

If you want to watch a video tutorial, go to www.6KeysPainFree.com. You'll be able to log on and access all the bonus material, including this trigger-point training. Or, you can read the instructions now and follow along. This can be applied to trigger points in any muscle of your body.

Sit at a table, take your dominant hand and lay it palm down on the table. Put your other hand on the top of the thickest part of your forearm to start exploring the extensor muscles there. The extensor muscles are the ones that lift your wrist and fingers. They get used a lot during the day especially if you work on computers.

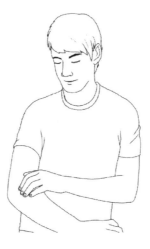

Lay your fingers on the skin of your forearm. Put your attention into the tips of your fingers. Run your fingers back and forth over your skin. You should be able to feel your skin gliding over your muscle fibres[5]. What the skin is gliding on is the underlying fascia.

Now, if you press a little deeper you should feel your forearm muscles. You'll feel them as individual sausage-like shapes running down your arm. As you go over them you'll be able to move backwards and forwards feeling each muscle. Now you can start pushing more firmly.

Keep your attention in the tips of your fingers, and as you move backwards and forwards you will feel a little tight band in one or more of the muscles. It feels something like a guitar string embedded in your muscle. As you put pressure on it, it will bounce back under your finger.

This tight band is your road to find the trigger point itself [6], because the trigger point will be somewhere along its length. Once your fingers are on the tight band you can now move up and down the band until you find a point that hurts as you push on it. This is the trigger point.

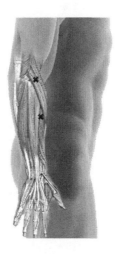

When you focus in on the trigger point you will feel a small lump or thickening in the muscle – at the most the size of the tip of your little finger. It's small, but as you press on it, because it's in the muscle, it may wobble around under your fingers. You have to pin it using two fingers to start accurately putting pressure on the point.

If you press quite hard on this point, it will feel sore and if it's particularly active you may notice the pain appears somewhere else as well. For this particular forearm trigger the pain usually runs down your forearm and you may feel it in your wrist or fingers.

Now that you're definitely on the trigger point, you're going to treat it and switch it off. This part is where many therapists take the 'no pain no gain' approach. They find the trigger point, and push on it with maximum pressure and pain.

Some people get a trigger point massage from an expert and it's absolute agony. The treatment may get them pain relief but they don't want to do it again. Treating a trigger point this way is unnecessarily painful and, in my experience, not the most effective course of action.

There's a completely different way to treat trigger points that is kinder to your body, and more effective. You're going to use ischemic pressure. Ischemic is a medical word meaning reduced blood flow. Remember, a trigger is caused by a grumpy nerve that's firing off an amplified pain message to keep the muscle in spasm. You are going to put this nerve to sleep.

Now you have your finger exactly on the trigger point, press just hard enough to make sure you're on the spot. You'll know you're on it because the pressure hurts. Then, reduce your pressure without moving your finger off the point. Reduce the pressure until you feel no pain.

This is the moment when you talk to the trigger point. You're talking to it in two ways – through your fingertips, and in your mind. You're using the mind-body connection to tell this nerve: "You don't need to protect me anymore. It's time to relax."

As you press on the trigger, practice your diaphragm breathing. Everything you are doing is designed to calm the area. Breathe, relax, and stay in this state for about thirty seconds. Then, slowly start to increase the pressure. You still haven't moved your finger a millimetre from the trigger point, but as you increase the pressure you will find it doesn't hurt.

Stay at this same pressure for thirty seconds then increase it again. Gradually, over two minutes, you will find you can push more and more and the trigger spasm simply melts away under your fingers. When this happens, you have painlessly turned off the trigger point. If you do feel pain at any time, reduce pressure until the pain recedes then slowly start to increase pressure again – staying below the pain threshold at all times.

That's the first part of the treatment. You can use this same technique for any other trigger in your body.

The second part of the treatment is stretching the muscle out to length. The tight band formed by the trigger has shortened the muscle. So once you've turned the trigger off you need to stretch out the tight band and return the muscle to normal mode.

Again, the best way to do this stretch is using a neuromuscular technique[7]. Everything in your body is related so you're going to combine several different systems to get the most relaxing stretch.

To do this, put your arm out straight in front of you. With your other hand, bend your wrist down towards the ground. Stretch until you reach the limit of comfort, then halt. Take a slow breath in while counting to six. As you breathe out, carry on counting.

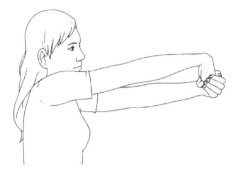

By the time you reach nine or ten, you will feel a remarkable thing happen. Your stretch limit will vanish and the muscle will effortlessly give just a little further. You will find there is a new zone of comfort where you couldn't go before. But you don't have to push anything as your muscles will gently glide further, and then reach this new limit.

Repeat the breathing and stretch process two or three times. This is how you switch off your triggers and reset your muscle length. At no stage do you need to cause pain or challenge your protective pain system.

There are other ways to treat trigger points and these include acupuncture and injections[8,9], however this book focusses on the optimal way for self-treatment.

*

Trigger points are an important piece of the chronic pain puzzle.[3] If your pain system has switched on trigger points, you now have the tools to very gently switch them off.

It's important to realise that without doing the mind-body practices from the earlier chapters, you will be treating trigger points without addressing the underlying cause. This means it's likely they'll return.

There is a dynamic tension between treating triggers and using mind-body techniques. On the one hand, treating triggers can be very effective for fast pain relief. But it requires you to put your attention onto the painful area, which is the opposite of what you do in mind-body techniques.

And so the difficult question arises: When do you use trigger treatment? And when do you use mind-body techniques? Because it is almost universal that trigger points *will* be present in an area where you have chronic pain.

So what are the guidelines? If you can use mind-body techniques and they totally abolish your pain, then you don't need to do anything else. If, however, you find there is still residual pain in the area, then you can treat those triggers with the understanding that treating the triggers will (in the long run) be helping your mind-body pain relief.

With this mindset, you can turn the attention you put on the painful area when you're treating trigger points into something positive. You're using the trigger treatment to relax your pain system, which will have a different effect in your mind.

When you combine ischemic trigger release with breathing and mind-body techniques, it has a powerful effect. For people who have difficulty doing just mind-body exercises, treating triggers is an effective way to interact physically with your pain system.

Now, we're going to erase the final doubts in your mind before plunging deep into the fascinating world of the subconscious.

11
Yes, But...

By now you understand amplified pain and how to treat it. This is where we get into the "Yes, but…" stage. What I mean is this: I see people every day in my clinic who have amplified pain. But when I explain what you now know, they say: "Yes, that's very interesting, but… I have: scoliosis/arthritis/damaged disc/spondylolisthesis/insert condition here." And you may be thinking the same thing.

The way to use this chapter is to skim till you find your particular diagnosis. We will only cover the most common ones. Before you read this book, it's likely you believed this diagnosis completely explained your pain.

You will discover:

1. The treatment options for your condition.
2. The pros and cons of these treatments.
3. Where pain amplification[1,2,3] fits into your picture.

You will get an idea of where you are in the transition between pain that is caused by physical damage and pain that is a malfunction in your pain system – and remember, it is not all or none.

Natural History

The first concept you need to understand is natural history[4]. This is what happens when you rely purely on the wonderful healing ability of your body, and do not seek intervention from health practitioners.

Every condition has its own natural history. It's useful because once you understand the natural history of your condition, you'll know whether your healing is progressing faster or slower than is normal.

Sometimes, people jump into serious treatments (like surgery) when all they needed was to wait for their body to heal.

Another thing that happens is you go to see someone for a problem, and they treat you long enough for your natural healing to kick in. You ascribe your getting better to their treatment, rather than the fact you got better naturally.

We're going to look at some of the common problems that begin people's descent into chronic pain, so you'll see where you sit in relation to the norm.

Damaged Disc in the Spine

The most common underlying cause of chronic back pain is a damaged disc in the spine.[26] The disc is a fascinating structure. It acts as a shock absorber between the vertebrae of your spine. There is a very strong disc wall (called the annulus), which is made up of 12 to 20 layers of collagen fibres that run at 90° angles to each other like a radial-ply tire. There are nerve endings only in the outer third of this wall. There are no blood vessels that run through the wall. Inside the disc there is a jelly-like material called the nucleus pulposis.

The interior of the disc gets its oxygen by diffusion and is metabolically incredibly slow. Things happen there at a rate similar to continental drift or glaciation. This is fine whilst everything goes well. However, once you damage the disc, healing will also be very slow.

So the timeframe to heal from a disc injury is measured in months, and sometimes up to two to three years. Understanding this is important because often people will rush into having treatments that all too often can interrupt this healing process.

When the disc is damaged, you will feel pain in the segment of the disc, but it can refer as an ache in a poorly-defined distribution. So a disc injury in the neck can ache into the arm and a disc injury in the back can ache into the buttock and leg.

The literature shows that, given time, about 70% of people will naturally get better following a disc injury.[4,11] I think this is very valuable information. The main reason people don't get better is that at some stage in the healing process, their pain system starts to malfunction. Then, even though the healing continues, the pain doesn't lessen. Now if you go and have surgery to your damaged disc (which is what you see on the MRI) your pain won't get better because the disc is no longer the primary cause of your pain.

It is important to note that the healing of the disc, even though effective, will never re-create the original pristine disc.

The disc will always look as though it is still damaged. This creates a real problem in trying to work out whether the pain is still due to the disc injury. Treating from the picture on the MRI will often not treat the problem[5].

There are two ways a disc can be injured. The first is the annulus may tear right through, so the jelly inside the disc (the nuclear pulposis) oozes out. This is called a disc prolapse. Now, because there is no blood supply to the nuclear pulposis, it is hidden from your immune system. This means that when it appears outside the disc, it is viewed by your body as a foreign substance. Therefore, your immune system immediately attacks it, and the area will become intensely inflamed. This can create a deep ache in your back.

The spinal nerves exit very close to the annulus of the disc, so they will often become inflamed as well. This creates a different kind of pain. Everyone knows the type of pain you get when you strike your 'funny bone'. It's a shooting electric pain down your arm into your little finger with associated tingling. This is because you have compressed the ulnar nerve in your arm and set off neuropathic pain – otherwise known as nerve pain.

When the nerve exiting your spine becomes compressed or inflamed, then you will have the same type of pain – a band of shooting, electric-type pain with tingling and numbness. The medical term for this pain is 'radicular pain' (pain arising from the nerve root).

The distribution of this pain is specific to each nerve. So a disc injury in your neck will refer down your arm. A disc injury in your thoracic spine will refer in a band around your back into your chest. And a disc injury in your lumbar (lower) spine will refer into your buttock and down your leg. This is called sciatica.

The natural history of a disc prolapse is that almost 90% of people[6] will recover within three to six months. However, if the pain does not resolve within this timeframe, then it can be a long-term problem. I lived with this pain for a very long time, but my injury had healed. The pain was from my malfunctioning pain system.

Radicular pain (pain from an inflamed nerve) is particularly difficult to treat. It responds poorly to most medications. There are, however, two treatments that tend to be more effective.

The first is to inject a long-acting cortisone preparation into the epidural space[7]. This is the space that surrounds the outer lining of the nerves. When the nerve is significantly inflamed, the cortisone will in effect 'put the fire out'. The cortisone will work for ten to twelve weeks, and will often give excellent pain relief for this period. This buys you time so you feel less pain while your body has the chance to heal.

The second treatment is to have the damaged disc trimmed back, and the disc material removed surgically. This can be done as a micro-discectomy [8] using new surgical techniques so it disrupts the area as little as possible. However, any surgery carries with it the extra risk [9] of a general anaesthetic, errors in the procedure, infection, plus epidural fibrosis.

Epidural fibrosis[10] is when your body lays down scar tissue in the epidural space. The scar tissue then behaves as scar tissue usually does, which is to slowly contract around the exiting nerve. This can produce long-term and very difficult-to-treat nerve pain. Therefore, I see surgery as a second line of treatment only to be resorted to if nothing else has worked.

The second type of disc injury is when the vertebral end-plate fractures. Even though this is bone, it is weaker than the disc wall (annulus). What happens here is the nucleus pulposus is squeezed up into the bone marrow inside the vertebra. The bone marrow has a huge blood supply, and the disc jelly that arrives turns on an intense immune system response.

The inflammation spreads into the disc and destroys it. This is called IDD – internal disc disruption[11], and is considered to be the most significant cause of chronic, unremitting low-back pain. This usually burns itself out in eighteen months to three years.

The final treatment of both of these conditions is to completely remove the disc. Then the surgeon may either replace the disc with a synthetic one, or fuse it. Disc replacement is a relatively new operation. The results from the first replacements were disappointing[12], because the discs didn't last. Newer discs look promising, but have only been in for a few years, so we don't know how long they will last.

The standard treatment after removing a disc has been to fuse the vertebrae above and below the disc[13]. They are fused by putting in bone (either from you, or a donor) and holding this bone in place with metal rods and screws. This takes many months to settle and changes forever the function of that segment of your spine. This can put increased pressure on the discs above and below the fusion site, which may then damage those discs, leading to a domino effect.

All of the treatments I've described have a certain success rate[14], but still there is a group of people who have ongoing pain. The damage to the disc may have cleared up. The disc may even have been removed and the spine fused – but the pain remains unchanged. Under these circumstances the primary problem lies in your pain system. Having further surgery or searching for some other magical cure is often an exercise in futility and frustration.

If you've had a disc injury, and you're past the normal recovery time, or you've had back surgery, and you've still in pain, then you need to look at pain sensitisation.

Other Spine Conditions

There are a number of other conditions that have splendid Greek names like spondylosis, spondylolisthesis and scoliosis. These terms are descriptive of observable changes on imaging (like x-ray or MRI). Spondylosis describes the set of changes that occur with normal use in your back – the 'wear and tear' of age. We've already discussed in chapter 6 that these changes do not predict pain at all.

Spondylolisthesis describes when one vertebra slips forward onto another. This occurs when there is a small break in the thinnest part of the vertebral arch (the pars interarticularis). You can be born with it or Spondylolisthesis can occur as a stress fracture from overuse. What then happens in most cases is your body lays down very strong scar tissue across the bony break, and stabilises the situation as best as it can.

Again there are many people with a stable spondylolisthesis who do not have pain[15]. If it is a high degree of slip or if it is increasing, then you need to be seen by a surgeon who is skilled and experienced in treating this kind of condition. The surgery will usually stabilise the slip but not put the bones back in its normal position. Therefore if a stable Spondylolisthesisis is present, it may not be the cause of your pain. Again, your pain may well be due to a pain system malfunction.

The same is true of scoliosis. Here, the spine when viewed from behind has an 'S' shape instead of being straight. There are many millions of people who have scoliosis without pain, in fact an excellent review article stated that the incidence of low-back pain is similar to the normal population[16]. Your body has a magnificent ability to adapt to changes, and it can certainly adapt to most scolioses.

Scoliosis has been comprehensively studied. It can become important when there is a significant degree of deformity, which occurs in a very small proportion of people. It is well known that if scoliosis occurs in a child, then it will worsen to a predictable degree as they go through their growth spurt in adolescence[17].

These children should be under the care of an orthopaedic surgeon who specialises in the assessment and treatment of scoliosis. In the vast majority of adults, the scoliosis is of a lesser degree and is not a significant problem. Many practitioners when they see these milder cases on x-ray or MRI scans will ascribe the pain to scoliosis. This is not true in most cases. Again, the underlying problem is usually your pain system, and requires you to do the treatments described in this book yourself.

Now we come to <u>arthritis</u>. This word has inspired fear and dread in so many people. I often get people in my consulting room who look at me with fear in their eyes and ask the question, "I hope it's not arthritis?"

Arthritis comes from two Greek words *'arth'* which means joint, and *'itis'* which means inflammation. So arthritis is purely a descriptive term meaning inflammation in a joint. When there is active inflammation in the joint, we are aware of it because the joint is swollen, hot, red, and painful. The inflammation may be just mild and slightly bothersome, or may be intense and extremely damaging. It depends on the cause of the inflammation itself.

There are times where the inflammation is part of an autoimmune disease like **rheumatoid arthritis**. Here your body's normal police force (the immune system) suddenly decides it's going to attack your own joint, and it does it very effectively. The inflammation is unceasing, very aggressive and damaging. In time the joint may end up completely destroyed.

When people think of arthritis, they usually think of people who have rheumatoid arthritis, where the joints are severely damaged and deformed. This type of arthritis is rare, and nowadays there are effective treatments that will stop the progression of the disease.

The most common type of arthritis is *osteoarthritis*. This is how it works; during your life, you may damage the cartilage of a joint. The cartilage is a beautiful, shiny, surface that acts as a frictionless shock-absorber between your bones. Cartilage, like your disc, gets its oxygen by diffusion, and therefore heals poorly. As the cartilage breaks down, your bones (which have a great blood supply) adapt to the damage, building bony buttresses so you can continue to use your joint.

The pictures of osteoarthritis you see on imaging are really these helpful adaptations. The important thing here is that an x-ray, CT scan or MRI showing osteoarthiritis does not equal pain. There are hundreds of millions of people in the world who have an x-ray, CT or MRI evidence of osteoarthritis in their joints yet do not have pain[18].

The important thing here is that there is a difference between spinal joints (vertebrae facet joints) and weight-bearing joints like your hip, knees or ankles. If there is significant osteoarthritis in the hip joint and you see it on an image, there is a much higher chance this is the cause of your pain. Fortunately, there is an excellent treatment – replace the joint.

Unlike major weight-bearing joints, spinal joint osteoarthritis has very little correlation with pain[19]. However, for those who do have pain emanating from the joint, there are also effective treatments.

At present the most-used treatment is anti-inflammatory medications, which can be helpful but do have side effects. The second treatment is to inject cortisone into the joint under direct imaging. This is effective but often only lasts as long as the cortisone (which is two to three months).

Whiplash describes a type of injury to your neck. In most cases somebody drives into the back of your car while you are stationary. Your body is pushed forward, but because you are restrained by the seatbelt you follow a slingshot movement upwards. Your head is free and therefore is flung backwards. If you were to look at the facet joint during a whiplash event, the lower portion is moving upwards with your body and the upper facet is coming backwards and down – so the two impinge upon each other.

This can cause damage within the joint, which then sends messages to the surrounding muscles to protect and they go into spasm. The literature shows the majority of people get better but it can take many months. There are a small proportion of people where they have long-term pain and for those there are treatments that are very effective[20].

One of these treatments is called radio-frequency neurotomy[20], where a probe is laid next to the nerve that supplies the joint and the nerve is microwaved (zapped).

This takes the pain message away and you do not feel pain until the nerve grows back, which is usually between nine to eighteen months. This breaks the pain cycle and often only needs to be done once. However, if your pain returns the process can be repeated. It is important to understand that this treatment is effective only for a small proportion of people with spinal injuries.

And now we come to the thorny issue of surgery. There is no doubt surgery is dramatic, and for those living with chronic pain, the surgeon seems like a knight in shining armour who is going to sweep in and make them better. Sometimes this is true, and for certain conditions surgery is superb. However, this is a much smaller list than most people think and hope.

Where surgery is best is the total hip joint replacement. The procedure was conceived about thirty years ago. The first prostheses were made of simple materials – stainless steel and plastic. When the first operations were done, surgeons told patients they would last maybe ten years. However, now it is recognised that over 90% last twenty years[21] and some of these hip replacements are still doing very well thirty years on.

What's interesting, the surgery involves cutting bone with saws, and complete destruction and removal of the old joint, and hammering in the prosthesis. It's a traumatic business.

Yet, when patients wake from surgery, most people feel relatively comfortable. They're walking within a short time, and within six weeks many are often pain free. This is surprising and wonderful.

So the results are splendid, and the surgery has become more slick, and has an astonishingly high success rate. 90-95% will be functioning at 10 years and 85% at twenty years.[22]

Knee and ankle joint replacements have had a rockier course, but the results have improved significantly. There is no doubt that for those with severely arthritic joints, the surgery outcomes[23] will be acceptable in the long term.

Unfortunately, the same is not true for spinal surgery[24]. The primary structure that causes much of spinal pain is the disc. Therefore using surgical reasoning, you must remove the disc. What we would like is then to replace the disc as we did with the joints. However, the technology is not there yet.

The final and significant difficulty with spinal surgery is that in the spine there are many segments close to each other. Each segment has a disc and two joints, plus many other possible pain-causing structures like ligaments, tendons and muscles. So it's very difficult to know which structure or segment is actually the cause of the pain. This is quite different from a hip joint where it is relatively easy to make that judgement.

So with spinal surgery the ongoing difficulty is knowing on which structure to operate. And this is why there are a proportion of people[25] who, after having the surgery, wake with exactly the same pain, plus the pain from the surgery itself. This is a difficult issue. For spinal surgery, this particular knight has tarnished armour. For this reason, it's a good idea to get two to three opinions from surgeons before operating.

Stenosis means narrowing. There can be stenosis of the central canal of the spine which causes pressure on the spinal cord. Also there can be stenosis of the side canals that cause pressure on the exiting nerve root. One of the better spinal surgeries is opening the space in the spine for nerves to run through. This usually gives good long term relief of nerve pain.

Now, I would like to touch on the various investigations that are available in an effort to figure out the cause of your pain. Each has strengths but also weaknesses.

X-rays

These have been around for 150 years. X-rays use high-energy ionising radiation, and when they are aimed at the body, they will pass through, only being slowed slightly by dense structures like bones. Therefore x-rays show bones beautifully and are very useful for looking at the skeleton. They are also cheap and widely available. However, the radiation is dangerous and is cumulative over your lifetime. Too much radiation increases the risk of cancer.

X-rays are used as a cheap screening tool, but lack the ability to look at soft tissues like discs, ligaments, tendons etc., which is where damage and pain often arises.

CT scan

CT scans also use x-rays. They show the bones and joints in exquisite detail, and soft tissues show up quite well. The problem with having a CT scan means you get a higher dose of radiation than a standard x-ray. One advantage is that using an advanced program, a computer can build a magnificent 3-D coloured image of your bones and joints.

Ultrasound Scans

These use high-frequency sound to create the image. It's a safe mode of investigation. Sound is beamed in a thin band into the body, and as it strikes tissues of different densities, is bounced back in an echo. The echoes are picked up by a transducer and fed into a computer to create a picture of the soft tissues in the area. This is an evolving technology, and modern ultrasounds show superb detail.

A huge advantage is that you can scan in real-time – looking at how muscles, ligaments and tendons glide as you're moving a limb. Ultrasounds show cysts and fluid extremely well and are useful in diagnosing possible causes of musculoskeletal pain.

MRI scans

For an MRI scan, you lie in a narrow tunnel surrounded by a very powerful magnet that changes polarity many times a second. This stimulates the atoms in your body to give off a signal. A computer creates a 3-D image and then makes very fine slices of that image. The resultant pictures show nerves, ligaments, tendons, blood vessels, bones and joints in superb detail.

At present this is the investigation of choice for many problems in the body. It is particularly good at viewing the disc and nerves of the spine. The problem is that an MRI only shows the anatomy. As we age, there are many 'abnormalities' picked up by the MRI, but they are merely the changes of wear and tear, and our bodies have adapted to them. This has created a major difficulty because it can be impossible to work out which (if any) of the abnormalities is actually causing the pain.

Functional Scans – MRI, Technetium and Sodium Fluoride

These have been devised to try to show abnormalities of function, not anatomy. They use either the oxygenation of blood or blood flow itself to show areas where there is increased metabolic turnover.

These show up as brighter-coloured areas on the scans – so-called 'hot spots'. The functional scan is then superimposed on a CT/MRI scan and you can then see one specific area highlighted. This technology is exciting and promises much; however, treatment of the highlighted area can still fail in a disappointing proportion of cases. These are definitely investigations for the future.

Blocking Nerves or Joints

Another way to work out which structure is causing your pain is to inject local anaesthetic either into a structure (like a joint) or around the nerves supplying that structure – thereby completely blocking messages coming to your brain.

These are called diagnostic blocks. In the spine, the most useful of these is to block the tiny nerves that supply the facet joints, especially in the neck and the lumbar spine. These are called medial branch blocks.

Best practice is that two medial branch blocks are done to reduce the chance of a placebo response. If these blocks are positive (meaning they have taken away your normal pain) then there is a procedure called a radio-frequency neurotomy that can literally microwave the nerve and give much longer pain relief. Unfortunately the nerve does grow back and therefore the procedure may need to be repeated. I do these procedures on a regular basis and, if best practice is followed, the results are excellent, with near complete pain relief in well over 75% of patients.[20] However, these procedures are only appropriate for a small proportion of the people I see.

The above was a brief summary of the conditions that occur alongside chronic pain. The difficulty is knowing how your pain (if any) is coming from these conditions. You can see the limitations of investigations in working this out.

This is why understanding and observing how your pain behaves is very helpful. You need to use the principles in this book to work out what is going on. While I recommend consulting competent medical professionals, in the end, you are the chief investigator for your own pain. You have the true inside information, and your health is more important to you than anybody else.

Now, we are going to venture into the shadowy realm of your subconscious. This is where you're going to uncover the deep drivers that stop your pain from getting better.

THE
FIFTH
KEY

12

The Underworld

"It is far more important to know what person has the disease, than what disease the person has."

~ Hippocrates

For the Fifth Key we need to go down into the murky underworld of chronic pain. We're going to look at the hidden forces that drive chronic pain in many people.

I should warn you before we start, this is challenging material. However, for many people this knowledge is the key to finally getting out of pain.

To introduce this topic, I'm going to share the story of a patient of mine. She was a very pragmatic lady, the wife of a farmer.

Meg came in, sat down and told me: "I have this burning pain. It came up out of nowhere and it affects both my arms and both my legs."

"That's quite an unusual pain," I said. "Can you give me a bit more detail?"

"Well, it's like a band of burning pain around my wrists and ankles. It's quite severe and gets worse when I lie down at night. It keeps me awake and quite frankly it's ruining my life."

We talked some more and then I asked an important question, one I find is always useful when I'm faced with a baffling situation like this. "Is there anything in your past that may have something to do with this pain, or is unusual?"

She sat for a moment in thought. Then her eyes opened a little wider. "You know in my twenties, about forty years ago, I became very depressed. I was committed to a mental hospital and was given electroconvulsive therapy for the depression."

"Yes, that is really interesting," I said.

Then she gasped. "I remember now. They used to tie me down with bands on my wrists and my ankles before doing the shock therapy. It was terrifying."

She sat there for a minute. Then she looked at me and said, "Do you think this could have something to do with my pain?"

"It seems highly likely," I said.

She then became thoughtful. "I remember that as a very dark time in my life."

"I think this is something from your subconscious that has resurfaced. Do you know of any reason why it's happening now?"

Together we explored this question and she couldn't think of anything that may have caused this memory to intrude on her life.

We talked over the concepts I'm about to share with you. In essence, her pain was coming from a traumatic past memory. It had been buried in her subconscious and had surfaced for an unknown reason. Instead of resurfacing as a memory though, it had surfaced as this mysterious pain, and now she needed to deal with it.

When I caught up with her three weeks later, the pain that had been with her many months before, had gone. In her search for a solution she'd seen three doctors and a neurologist. None of them could make any sense of her strange pain. But it melted away once she found the genesis of it in her own mind. In this chapter we're going to explore what Meg did, and how you can do the same.

Welcome to the fascinating world of your subconscious mind. To take the next step into this realm you need to meet two people. The first is Dr Sigmund Freud. He was one of the original great psychiatrists. Freud brought forward the idea that we have a conscious mind, which we are all aware of. However there is a whole other world deep inside us, which is our subconscious mind. This subconscious mind is, by definition, hidden.

If you are aware of something then it is part of your conscious mind. Nothing in your subconscious mind is visible to you. According to Freud it is a strange and sometimes dangerous place.

Freud wrote many things about the subconscious mind, and a lot of them were concerned with sex. This isn't what we're going to be looking at. We're most concerned with his original work and the concept of a hidden part inside our mind. The burning pain in Meg's wrists and ankles was a dramatic example of the power of this hidden, subconscious mind.

The second person I'm going to introduce you to is a fascinating doctor by the name of John Sarno. Dr Sarno was a pain physician practicing in New York City in the 1980s and 90s. He had a conventional practice, which he set up along the lines of most pain clinics. However he found the results he was getting were not very good (like most standard pain clinics of the day).

It was while running his pain clinic that Sarno had a stunning insight into why common treatments for chronic pain were not working. The reason people were not getting better was because doctors were treating the wrong thing.

Sarno had studied Freud and the subconscious mind. He brought forward the theory that most (if not all) chronic pain was being driven by the subconscious.

This was a revolutionary idea (and still is not accepted by mainstream medicine). However, Sarno fully committed to it. He had originally run a multi-disciplinary clinic with people who did physical rehab and other modes of treatment. When he decided to pursue his theory, Sarno dismissed everyone from his clinic who didn't work on the psychological aspect of pain.

What he found was fascinating. A proportion of people who didn't get better with any other methods had remarkable success with his treatment.

Sarno's thinking was way ahead of its time. It's only recently that medical science has started to recognise the importance of the mind-body connection and its powerful effect on chronic pain. His concept may not be able to explain all chronic pain. However there's great value in understanding the mind-body connection. It's another tool you can use to reset your pain system and return to pain free life.

Your Personality

All of us are governed by larger patterns in our self. We're mostly unaware of them, but when we do talk about them, we give them names like our personality traits or character. These traits are driven by deep-seated beliefs living inside our minds. What most people in chronic pain are unaware of is that when certain traits occur strongly they can feed your pain.

Over fourteen years running a pain clinic I've met many people with chronic pain. And a large proportion of them have the traits I'm going to describe. It's not just my observations though. The literature on chronic [1,2,3,4] pain also supports this.

There are two traits that stand out. The first is perfectionism. People with chronic pain tend to set very high standards for themselves. They feel bad about themselves if they're not able to meet these standards.

How does perfectionism begin? A common scenario is when an important person in your childhood praises you for a job well done. You do something for this person and they say to you, "You did that job *so* well. You are such a good boy/girl because you did the job so well."

Now, the first clause in that last sentence – "you are good person because you did a good job" – may or may not have been said. But as a child you made the connection: being a good person equals doing a good job. You've learnt the only way for you to be good is for you to do the job perfectly. The flip side of this is: if you don't do a good job, you're not a good person.

This belief system has certain benefits. If you follow it you become very trustworthy. You're always going to go the extra mile and do a job incredibly well, and this will take you far in your work and your relationships.

But it carries with it an incredible burden. The dark side of perfectionism is that inside you, there lives a slave driver who is always demanding more. Even if you're tired, exhausted, and in pain, you are going to push yourself to do a job to your exacting standards.

Perfectionism also causes suffering because if you want everything to be perfect, you are always aiming for something out of reach. No matter how good a job you do, it's never perfect. This creates growing pressure inside you. Eventually this pressure will cause a breakdown – either in your mind or body[5].

The second common trait of people in chronic pain is self-sacrifice[6,7]. Someone with this character trait is always out there helping people and putting others first. They are caring and nurturing, but don't take time to look after themselves. For a self-sacrificing person, being 'good' and taking care of other people's needs *always* comes before fulfilling their own needs.

Like perfectionism, this martyrdom has a good side of unselfishly serving others. But it has a dark side too. When you're always putting others first, you're constantly denying your own needs. And over time there is a hidden cost.

What is the root of this trait? Looking after your own needs last comes from low self-esteem. Deep down, you don't believe you are deserving of nurturing and putting yourself first.

Self-esteem is a mysterious thing that occurs when you're very small. Early on, you either believe that you're ok, or you believe you are not ok. It has nothing to do with how intelligent or talented you are. It has everything to do with a belief you hold deep down – often without being aware of it.

These two personality traits – perfectionism and self-sacrifice – are incredibly powerful drivers of your behaviour. And they will, over time, push you towards the edge of a cliff.

There've been times when I've been in my clinic with a patient and I can see them talking themselves out of doing the things they need to do in order to get better. For some reason, making their health the priority goes against a deep-seated belief that is invisibly shaping their decisions.

So perfectionism and self-sacrifice are two character traits that often underlie chronic pain. Before we look at how to remedy this, let's review the other factors that contribute to ongoing pain.

Remember the study[22] showing the dramatic rise of chronic pain in chapter 6? Here's another cause: the civilisation we have made moves faster than ever before.. Job security is a vanishing concept. Competition is higher as we are now a global economy and outsourcers can compete for office worker's jobs all over the world. The speed of technological advance means the job you're doing may not even exist in five years' time.

If reading the last paragraph makes your blood pressure rise right now, you're not alone. In fact, people in the developed world work longer hours, have less job satisfaction and are less secure than people twenty years ago[8,9]. All these pressures around work create stress. And unrelenting stress takes a toll on the body, making the descent into chronic pain more likely.

With all these forces in play, let's return to Sarno's theory of chronic pain and the subconscious. There is a division in our mind that separates the things we are conscious of, and the vast submerged subconscious. Until now we've worked in the domain of the conscious mind. All the mind-body techniques in chapter 7 are in your conscious mind. It's now time to venture into the realm of the subconscious.

The subconscious mind is very powerful[10]. Many of our thoughts and actions are guided by the subconscious, though we are unaware of it. It's the area we access when we dream. The language of your subconscious – like the language of dreams – is metaphorical and symbolic.

To understand how pain may be caused by your subconscious mind, let's imagine what could lie in the subconscious. Freud [11], Jung and many others spoke of archetypes living within our subconscious mind. These archetypes are the basic building blocks of character, existing in all cultures.

The three primary archetypes Freud believed drove the subconscious[11] are the adult, the parent and the child. The child is also known as the 'id', and it is the child we are particularly interested in. This small child lives in all of us. Like a real toddler it is self-centred, irresponsible and irrational. It wants to be satisfied now, never later.

The problem is that as an adult, the demands of the child are being constantly ignored. You have to deny them in order to be a functioning grown up. While the child or id in you may want to eat ice cream and watch TV all afternoon (until something else strikes its fancy) the adult in you knows you have to go back to work.

When you deny the id's desires – all day, every day, for years – your inner child has a tantrum from hell. According to Freud, your inner child manifests a constant, permanent rage, and this rage lives within your subconscious mind. This rage fills the whole of your subconscious mind – paints it red.

Most people who hear this theory respond by saying, "Yes, that's interesting, but I'm not an angry person." The point to make here is you're not aware of this rage. It lives in your subconscious, and so by definition you can't be conscious of it.

This also shows why what we're exploring is a theory – it is impossible to prove. However, by accepting it as a working hypothesis, and questioning how it could affect your thoughts and emotions, many people have had breakthroughs with their chronic pain.

So how could all this rage come to live in your subconscious mind, and you be unaware of it? The answer lies in the act of repression. In the hidden division of your mind, time doesn't pass like it does in your conscious mind. Time stands still, and this is key to understanding repression and subconscious rage.

Imagine you were three years old and someone gave you the most delicious ice cream. But just as you were about to take your first bite, a horrible older sibling grabbed it and ran off. Any three year old in this situation would feel as if their whole world has come to an end. If this were you, you would feel the most intense emotions – sadness, rage and loss. And these emotions would be so powerful you could not cope with them.

When you're faced with an unbearable situation, your conscious mind does something interesting. It calls on your subconscious mind to help. To escape the terrible emotions, you repress the painful experience. You push it from your conscious mind into the subconscious mind. But remember, time passes differently there. So while you're no longer aware of the pain, loss and anger, in that timeless place they still live, suspended in amber. Memories lie dormant but unchanged, with all their attendant fury, hurt, and other negative emotions you weren't able to handle at the time.

As you go through life, all the painful experiences you didn't have the ability to cope with are repressed. Some of them weren't so terrible (like a stolen ice cream) but you couldn't cope with them because you were very young. Other experiences may be truly traumatic, like abuse or losing a loved one. There is a high correlation between early trauma and chronic pain[12,13,14].

All your repressed experiences join the sea of rage in your subconscious. In the picture Freud paints, your subconscious is a dark and dangerous place, full of things that scare you and need to be locked safely away.

If we now put all the pieces together, what you get is an intolerable situation. Outside, pressures are increasing, pushing you into uncertainty and stress. Inside, your perfectionism is driving you to strive for an unattainable goal. You keep putting others needs before your own, further enraging the child inside you, which wants its own desires met. And you need to keep striving and denying yourself because you believe deep down you're not ok. And even deeper inside, in your subconscious, live threatening experiences from your past, sunk in a sea of rage.

It's a dark picture, and if even part of it were true, you can see how this would drive anyone to breaking point.

Now, here comes Sarno's insight. What he states is that on some level, your conscious mind knows about the scary things repressed in your subconscious. And knowing this, your conscious mind fears that with all these other pressures pushing you, the repressed emotions are going to come into your conscious mind. The line dividing the two minds is wearing thin and the sea of violent emotions is starting to rise.

To control the situation your conscious mind does something remarkable. It creates a diversion. One that is guaranteed to obsess you and take up all your attention.

And the perfect diversion? You turn on chronic pain, either somewhere in your body – or all over your body. Sarno called this condition 'TMS' (tension myoneural syndrome) and related it to a lack of oxygen in the muscles.

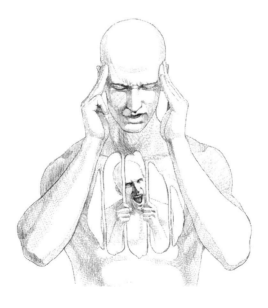

With modern neuroscience we can attribute a different mechanism to chronic pain. We can now see the process of pain amplification in the nerve synapse. By altering the neurotransmitters up and down your spinal cord, your pain system can create and amplify any sensation up to the level of pain[15,16,17].

Sarno's wonderful insight is how certain personality traits combined with stress and repressed emotions create an intolerable situation. As a desperate measure to try to cope, *you create your own pain as a diversion*. You're not doing this on purpose, and you're not doing this consciously. It is a survival strategy of your mind when it believes it has nowhere else to turn. To escape overwhelming pressure, you unknowingly create a monster that's worse than the one you were running from.

This is what happened with Meg. Her memories of shock therapy in her early twenties were so traumatic she had suppressed them deep in her subconscious. At the time this was the only way she could deal with the situation. Even forty years later, her conscious mind still perceived the memory as so dangerous that it chose to manifest physical pain as a diversion rather than have her become aware of it.

Meg went back to that time in her mind, and saw herself as she had been – young, depressed and powerless. And now she was a happily married grandmother who was confident in herself and her place in the world. This mature Meg could talk to her subconscious and reassure it that everything was safe, and she didn't need to be protected from traumatic memories any more. She told her mind 'I do not need to create this pain any more. I am safe.' By disarming this memory, she was able to lay it to rest and her pain also disappeared.

To support this theory of pain as a diversion, recent studies have shown[18,19] that as pain becomes chronic, it activates a different part of your brain – the part that also processes emotion. This means chronic pain is totally different from acute pain. And in treating it you also need to address your underlying emotional health.

If this theory resonates with you (and many people I talk to find it does) then what can you do about it?

There are several approaches I've seen work. The first most important step is to do what Meg did with the burning pain in her wrists and ankles. She clearly saw the link between her present pain and a traumatic past experience, and realised some part of her was creating the pain.

The next step is to talk to your brain. If we accept Sarno's theory, your pain was originally created by your mind trying to help you. Now you need to let this same part of your mind know its help is no longer needed, or at least not in this way. This may sound too simplistic to work, but in doing this you are interfering with the process that turned on the pain in the first place.

To do this, make a practice of sitting each morning and evening in a quiet place. Begin your session by becoming still and telling your mind: 'Whatever you're trying to distract me from, the pain you're creating is ten times worse. Let's look at this suppressed memory you're afraid of. If it's something from when I was young, I'm sure I can deal with it now.

'If it turns out to be something seriously traumatic and I've suppressed it, then I'll get whatever help I need. But first you need to stop creating this pain because it's ruining my life.'

Once you enter this part of your journey there are as many possible outcomes as there are people. For example this is what happened for me.

I discovered this concept having struggled for many years with low back pain and sciatica. As part of my treatment, every night and every morning I would close my eyes and talk to my subconscious.

'I know that my subconscious has many hidden, dark secrets. I am tired of this pain and don't need it. Therefore bring it on! Lay before me every repressed memory I have and I will either deal with it by myself or I'll get help.'

I waited and waited. Each time I did this, nothing of real note popped up in my mind. At the same time I was addressing the reactive part of my pain, and learning how to change my reaction to spam pain messages. Doing all these techniques together, my pain melted away over two to three months. This pain has never returned.

I discovered no deep, dark, terrifying repressed memories, but I believe this practice was an important part of getting better. However, some people I've worked with did discover painful repressed memories.

Jack was a hard-working professional in his early-60s. He had lived with chronic pain in his neck, radiating up into his head and across his chest. He described the pain as a "pressure feeling, sort of constricting". He often felt extreme anxiety when the pain was most severe. It had been present for about sixteen years and he had found that it was interfering both with his personal and professional life to an increasing degree.

I felt this was an unusual quality of pain and so introduced the concept of repressed emotions in his subconscious being a possible cause of chronic pain. He looked at me quizzically and then smiled. "Okay, I will talk to my subconscious..."

I saw him a month later and he recounted this story. He had followed the practice of asking his subconscious every morning and every night. On the tenth night he felt the hair rise on the back of his neck, broke into a sweat and found himself hyperventilating. He said it was as though the train was coming in to a station – at first tiny and then growing in his mind. The memory arrived. He was a small child. There was a large man with his arms around his neck squeezing and whispering in his ear, "If you tell anyone, I will have to kill you." This man then proceeded to rape him.

This terrifying event was repeated over a few months and then the man disappeared. Jack thought he may have been some relative staying in the house, but could not remember his name or even clearly see his face. Whilst telling me this story, tears rolled down his cheeks and he was wracked with sobs. I introduced him to a superb psychologist and he got help to heal this trauma. As part of his therapy, he continued to explain to his subconscious that he no longer needed the pain and indeed his pain stopped.

These are two extremes. Many other people have found repressed memories that are not as traumatic, but seemed to underlie or drive their chronic pain.

The next part of coming to the place where you can stop this pain is to go back to chapter 2 and review how amplified pain works. You need to accept amplification as the cause of your pain. This means believing there's actually not much wrong with your body, and you can begin to resume your normal activities.

There is a caveat for resuming normal activities which we'll cover in the rest of this chapter – it has do with perfectionism and your inner slave driver. But the most important thing now is to accept your chronic pain problem lies not in the structures of your body but in the workings of your pain system.

What you have now is an explanation for why your pain amplification got turned on. It's an explanation many people have found illuminating and they've seen in themselves the intolerable situation that drives it.

For many people chronic pain – unwelcome as it is – was the final desperate call from a body and mind pushed beyond all limits. So to truly heal, you need to look at the mental and emotional causes, not just the physical.

Many people I've worked with have also made sweeping changes to their lifestyle in order to heal from pain. They've been able to see clearly how the way they approached their work and relationships was putting far too much pressure on themselves. They've had to learn to put themselves first, and listen carefully to the small voice inside them that tells them what they really want in life. In essence, to heal the internal causes of chronic pain, many people have to learn once again to unconditionally love and accept themselves.

I believe all of us come into this world as perfect beings. In the process of learning to fit into at times an insane world, we've all made adjustments to our essential nature. We've all learned to hide or deny parts of ourselves we feel won't be accepted by others. When we take this too far, the psychological pain this causes can end up manifesting as physical pain. Perhaps our mind feels this physical pain is easier to deal with than pain to your heart (in some cases it may well be right).

The process of relearning to love and accept yourself, with all your attendant foibles, vulnerabilities, and quirks is a beautiful part of healing from chronic pain. And one that will enrich your whole life, not just your physical health.

Trish was a sixty-two-year-old office administrator who was due to retire in three years. She presented with chronic pelvic pain for which she had had a hysterectomy and removal of her ovaries. Unfortunately, this had not improved her pain at all.

She described a deep ache that was always there, and was much worse at work, when she went to the toilet, and when she had sex. She found the pain hard to cope with, and recognised she had become increasingly depressed. She was alternately distant and irritable towards her partner at home, and frustrated with her workmates.

She told me she felt her life closing in around her, and that she had no one to confide in who understood her.

In talking with her, we uncovered dreams she'd left behind in the daily grind of work, raising a family, and life. Though it had seemingly nothing to do with her pain, I encouraged her to live out some of those things she'd dreamed of doing.

She started singing lessons, which she'd always wanted to do. She reached out to her mother, whom she'd had a rocky relationship with, and was able to forgive her. She bought a dog and started walking it with her partner each day.

She practiced the breathing from chapter 9, and gradually as other parts of her life improved, and her emotional barriers came down, she was able to express more of her creative self. Her pain went away.

At this stage, some of you reading this may have the following objections:

Are you trying to tell me my pain is all in my head? Do you not believe my pain is real?
Are you saying I need to go to see a shrink to get rid of my pain?

My answer to the first two questions is: no, of course not. Any pain you feel is real pain, regardless of the cause or whether it's paired with physical damage or not.

My answer to the third question is that in most cases, this exploration of your subconscious doesn't uncover anything that would require you see a psychologist. In some cases it does, but mostly it doesn't. If you don't uncover any suppressed memories that may explain your pain, that's fine. Don't get obsessed with searching your past. This exploration is just another possible pathway that is meaningful for some people but not everyone.

The question of emotional pain being translated into physical pain brings up the findings of functional MRIs I mentioned earlier[20]. Brain scans show that once pain becomes chronic, emotions and chronic pain are processed in the same part of your brain.

If you were so beaten down by life your mind chose pain over facing suppressed emotions, is it now possible you may need to change your relationship with yourself to heal your body and mind?

For many people, getting out of chronic pain also means changing your beliefs about yourself. It is a process of learning to love and nurture yourself. People I've talked with discover they need to stop pushing themselves all the time. They learn to accept themselves, even when they aren't able to do a job 'perfectly'.

They learn to forgive themselves when they fall short of an impossible goal instead of judging themselves harshly as they would in the past. Those who truly dive into this new challenge meet themselves in a new way, and awaken a part of themselves they may have lost years ago – the part that loves themselves unconditionally, not for what they can do, but for who they are.

If you can see in yourself some of the characteristics I described above, here are some broader practices people have found helpful for diffusing the driving traits of perfectionism and self-sacrifice.

The first thing to recognise is it's hard to give up the habits of perfectionism and being driven. Many people who have these traits recognise they are the secret to their success. It's hard to abandon what was a winning formula, even if it's now causing you pain.

Being a perfectionist may have helped you to succeed in your career, your personal life and made you a trusted and respected person. Telling your inner slave driver to take a back seat can be harder than quitting smoking. For many people, it feels "wrong".

Changing the habits of a lifetime will always feel wrong. Trying something different can be uncertain and uncomfortable, even scary. However, unless you adopt a new mode of being in your life, you're doomed to repeat the same mistakes that got you into this trouble in the first place.

One exercise I've found helpful is something I discovered as a young doctor. I would often be racing into emergency situations, full of caffeine and low on sleep. In those days trainee doctors often worked hundred-hour weeks in the hospital. The situations I would land in were often tense and full of stressed people.

I trained myself to take a couple of breaths – in slowly, and out slowly. During this single breath, I would feel the gift of relaxation that comes every time you breathe out. I would remind myself that I could only do my best. And there is a place where doing your best ends and the outcome begins. You do your best, and the outcome from this place onwards will be what it will be.

Going into that situation I knew that I would do everything I could within my sphere of influence. But where that sphere of influence ended, was also where my responsibility ended. One of the biggest sources of stress is trying to affect things that are outside your sphere of influence. Working as a doctor in a hospital, there were many things outside my sphere of influence, including whether the patient lived or died. We would all do our very best, but if it was that person's time to go, they would go.

One question I get people to ask themselves in a stressful work situation is: "Will anyone die if X doesn't happen?"

Unless you work in emergency care or disaster rescue, the answer is often no; which helps to put things a little more in perspective. But even if lives are on the line, taking a few breaths to collect yourself and remind yourself that all you can do is your best, is very freeing. It will help you do your work better, and more importantly, it will allow you to only take responsibility for the things which truly are your responsibility.

Catastrophizing and the Cascade

Another frequent method employed by the inner slave driver is the cascade. You may not recognise it because it hides under a film of anxiety. Here is an example of how it works: one morning, it looks like you going to be late for work.

The traffic is slow, and you got out of the house five minutes later than usual because you were helping your kids get ready for school. Stuck in traffic there is really nothing you can do to get to work quicker. But the threat of being late lingers around you, causing you to feel bad. In fact you feel awful. You feel anxious, jittery, and your heart is beating uncomfortably fast in your chest.

This is where questioning the cascade comes in. If you pause for a moment you will find that underneath the veneer of anxious, bad feelings are a group of racketeer thoughts.

They've gathered like the proverbial village gossips and are adding to the cascade. The cascade is an imagined series of follow-on events that stem from the situation you're currently in.

The cascade sounds like this: 'I'm going to be late for work. Everyone will look at me as I come into my desk and they will know that I'm late. Because of this, they will think I am a bad worker, and a bad person. My boss will see me coming in late, and will think I don't take my job seriously. Then, when the next series of restructuring takes place, she will put me at the top of the list of people to be made redundant. And so I will lose my job, and I will not be able to find another one for many, many months. And because of this I won't be able to pay the mortgage on my house, and I'll have to sell it at a huge loss. And then I'll be in debt and without a job, and my kids will go and stay with my sister, my mother-in-law will say 'I told you so', and everyone in my family will view me as a failure, and the rest of my life will be awful, forever, and I'll never be happy ever again.'

I think you'd agree this is a fairly far-fetched series of events. But if you dig a little bit into the thoughts nattering away underneath your anxiety as you sit in traffic, you may find something quite close to this.

And this represents a golden opportunity. This is where you can step in and ask yourself, "Is this true?" and "Is this even likely?"

Because most of the time no one really knows or cares if you are late. They are too worried about themselves. They are caught up in their own cascade of worries and unrealistic fears. And why would you lose your job over being late? And even if you did, I'm sure you could do some temporary work until you found a job that really suited you. And even if the very worst scenario came about – the deepest fear underneath it all that you would never be happy ever again – is simply not true.

We know this because there have been studies on people who have had very serious life changes like becoming a paraplegic. A year later most people report about the same level of happiness. Paradoxically, this is also true of people who win the lottery[21].

The point is, the secret fears that drive perfectionism don't need to be so secret. You can pull them out into the light of day and ask them to please explain themselves. It is highly likely they won't be able to – not convincingly anyway.

Getting into this habit of questioning what is driving the negative emotions in your life is very liberating. It will help you in the next step.

And this next step is practising something called pacing.

The reason you need to practice pacing is in order to break the *Boom and Bust cycle*. This cycle is one of the hidden patterns keeping people in chronic pain. I have had cases when this alone has been enough to get someone out of years of pain and back to their normal life.

Here's how the Boom and Bust looks. Supposing you're a 'type A' person. You take your responsibilities seriously. You can't bear to leave a job until it's up to your high standard, let alone leave it half done.

But your pain has flared lately, leaving you so incapacitated you're unable to do any of your usual chores. So you rest, creating a growing to-do list in your head. Then one morning – miraculously – you wake and feel pretty good. In fact, you're feeling positively energetic.

So you mentally dust off your list of Important Things That Must Be Done, and set to doing them. It's mid-afternoon before you pause for a breath, and as you go to sit down, you do so with the awful slow-dawning realisation that you have overdone it.

You've pushed your just-recovered body too far, and the growing ache in your back is your body presenting the bill. The flare in your pain system is so bad you end up having to rest and take pain meds for the next four days, unable to do much more than drag yourself through the day and review your to-do list with despair. Until one day you wake up, and you feel pretty good…

Can you recognise this cycle in your own life? Many people I talk to in my pain clinic repeat this exact pattern. For some of them it's household chores. For others it's hobbies or the sports they love. Behind this pattern are two things: the need to do a good job (and thus be a good person), and the clinging-on to how things 'should' be.

Let's look at the 'should be' part of this equation. If you were an active person before your pain started, then there's a part of you still mourning the loss of that identity. And another part is full of anger, frustrated at not being able to do the things you used to do. Things 'should' be different.

The problem is if you're unable to let go of how things 'should' be then you're blocked from trying a different stance. It's also easy to remember the time before you had pain as an ideal period where you never had any troubles. If you could only get rid of your pain, things would be perfect again.

I'm sorry to say that when you get rid of your pain you will still have problems. They will be different problems, more interesting ones perhaps. But right now, caught in this current situation, you need to learn the lessons of this challenge. You ended up in this predicament partly because you were doing things in a way that pushed you over the edge of a cliff. There's no blame or judgement attached here. Damning yourself because you're in pain is not going to help.

However, there is hard-won knowledge you can seize from this situation and bring with you as you move forward. This knowledge will help you live a better life in the future even as you return to pain-free living.

So, if you are to let go of how things 'should' be, and recognise the inner slave driver, what do you do differently on the day when you wake up feeling good, with an enormous list of things you want to get done?

First, know for a fact that even if you only do one item on the list no one is likely to die. Take a deep breath and sit with that thought. As you release your breath, release the tension and compulsion you feel as you look at your list.

Next, as you start the first item, you're going to practice pacing.

Here is how to pace. Before you start your first job, divide it into four to six small parts. As you finish each division, stop. Take a breather, have a cup of tea, and congratulate yourself on how well you've done that section, and how well you're practicing pacing. Allow yourself to feel satisfied in the moment, with the world and your place in it.

Then, *and only then*, ask yourself: 'How am I feeling? Do I still feel full of energy? Do I still feel completely well?' If the answer is yes (and no deluding yourself please) then you are allowed to move to the next section of the job. If you feel even a small twinge, a warning sign you may be tiring, then down tools. You've done plenty for today.

When you stop booming and busting, a surprising thing happens. Instead of a mammoth effort (the boom) and then a flare that knocks you out for days (the bust) your time of feeling well starts to grow. If you do as I described and stop as soon you start to tire, you may find the next day you're still feeling pretty good. So you can do a little more.

I had one lady come into my clinic who had had significant widespread body pain for years. She had been to multiple clinics and seen many experts. It turned out her mother had also suffered from pain in the same way. When I described this boom and bust pattern I could see the recognition of it in her eyes.

"That's *exactly* how I work," she said.

Over a period of several months she practiced pacing her work. And to everyone in the clinic's delight, she was able to finally leave her pain behind. So pacing is a powerful tool.

The other way in which people drive themselves to their detriment is with self-sacrifice. This one can be hard to face. Again, it may form an important part of your identity. Helping others may give you joy and meaning. However, if it is coming at the price of your health, you need to ask yourself if it is really helping.

Think of the warnings we all ignore before our plane takes off: "In the event of cabin pressure dropping, an oxygen mask will come down from the ceiling." And here's the crucial part: "You need to put your own oxygen mask on first before you try to assist anyone else."

If you are trying to cope with chronic pain, how much are you able to help others anyway? Is it not more generous in the long run to put yourself first, get better, and then look after others?

Examining yourself to see if putting others first is costing you, is something only you can do. It requires insight and asking some hard questions. If your primary identity is being a caregiver, and you have difficulty with being looked after by others, then this is something you need to look at.

Because while you may hide from yourself, in the end your body and mind will find a way to help you, and it may not be a way you like. If you are always saying 'yes' to things you really want to say 'no' to, what better way to escape this than having a condition where you are forced to say no?

This is delicate territory to approach. And because we're having this conversation in the mode of text on a page, I cannot approach it as sensitively as I would in person. When I discuss this with someone in a consultation, the objections I address are: "You mean I'm making this up?" And: "So you think it's my fault I'm in pain?"

And the answers are no, I don't think you're making it up, and no, I don't think it's your fault. But, you are more powerful than you know, and in this circumstance you have the power to change how your pain system reacts. Gently, over time. Without self-recrimination or anger.

The interaction between your conscious mind, your subconscious mind and your personality is a very powerful thing. When you start looking to this quarter for the solution to your pain, you may be surprised at what insights emerge. Often it's the obvious things that hide in plain view – things you really knew all along – that make the biggest difference in your life.

For some, pain is an unwelcome wake-up call to look at parts of their life they have covered up. Setting your life back in balance is part of healing, and a process that can make you better than before.

THE SIXTH KEY

13
Move Like a Child

When part of your body hurts, the first thing you figure out is which movements cause pain. Depending on where you hurt (whether it's your shoulder, leg, hip, or back) you'll start unconsciously changing your movement to avoid causing yourself pain. These unnatural movements include things like limping, holding yourself to one side, restricting your normal range of movement and guarding yourself constantly.

This adaptation is fine when you're injured and your pain system is functioning correctly. It's how you keep from making your injury worse. After some time, your injury heals, the pain goes away and you return to your normal movements.

However, when your pain doesn't go away, most people carry on making their unusual movements to avoid using the parts that hurt. In my years as a pain physician, I have seen some astonishing adaptations that people make in the hope they'll be able to avoid their terrible pain.

There is a problem with this. If you've been in pain for months or years, it's highly likely the original cause of pain has healed. You're now left with pain caused by a malfunctioning pain system. And now, *you've unknowingly linked the unnatural movement to your amplified pain.* It's become part of the Reactive pain pattern we talked about in chapter 4, and your unnatural movement now feeds the pain cycle.

This means there are two things going against you. First, you're moving in a way your body was never designed to move. Often this alone is enough to generate pain. But secondly, as you make the unnatural movement, it links in and winds up your pain-system malfunction, sometimes prolonging it indefinitely.

For example, suppose you get pain whenever you get out of a chair. You adapt your movement to minimise the pain, but it still hurts. Now every time you get out of a chair, you're tensing your muscles and moving very slowly and awkwardly. As this unnatural movement becomes habitual, something else occurs that is very powerful. You start to anticipate the pain before you make the movement. This turns on your pain amplifiers in a conditioned response. You've virtually guaranteed the movement will be painful.

Over time, the abnormal way of moving becomes a habit (see chapter 8). The habitual-movement pattern is taken over by a deeper structure in your brain – the basal ganglia[1,2], which resides in the lizard brain or midbrain. New movement patterns are difficult, but if you do them often enough, they reach the point when you no longer have to actively think to perform them. This process occurs with all movement patterns, from the time we learnt to roll over as a little baby lying on our backs, up until today. If you're learning a useful movement pattern, it means you can do it more efficiently and your brain uses less energy. This frees you up to do other things at the same time. It's how we can drive, talk and do our hair all at once (not recommended). But the unnatural movements you've adopted are now an invisible habit that prolongs your pain.

A most interesting thing happens when I help people in my pain clinic return to natural movement. They find they're able to go back to a better way of moving, and it no longer hurts. They may get the odd twinge as they transition, but after a few days of moving naturally they are able to rediscover relatively pain-free movement.

When you were injured, the pain was like a fiery cage around you. You moved less and less and trimmed the edges of what you did in order to stay 'safe'. But your body has healed. It has an amazing·capacity to get better from even the most serious injuries. The door to the fiery cage is now open. What you now need to do is brave the heat and get out of the cage.

You have mind-body techniques to turn down your amplified pain. Now it's time to challenge your pain system by moving the way you used to. Like a bird that has been caged for a years, it may take you some time to even notice the door is open. It will take courage to venture outside the cage. But when you do so, you will discover a new freedom and joy in movement you had long forgotten.

I've seen this happen many times for people within a twenty-minute session in my clinic. And I was able to work this same transformation for my back pain. So if you're ready to restore pain-free movement, let's get started.

*

So how do you regain your natural-movement patterns? We're going to explore how to do this with some common movements and postures. Many people find these examples are relevant to their movement.

Action Step #1

The first step is training your observational powers to see where you have adopted unnatural movement. Each time you notice yourself moving in a weird way to avoid anticipated pain – stop. Make a mental note of the movement, and then experiment. See if you can make the movement in a more relaxed way. Try breathing calmly as you move. Take time to remember how you used to make this movement, then search for the simplest and most efficient way to do it.

Ask your family and friends if they notice you moving strangely. It's even worth asking someone to film you with their cellphone, so you can see what you're doing. You may find by doing this exercise, you end up moving better than you did before your pain started.

Action Step #2

The second step is constantly reminding yourself that the pain message you're getting is not related to physical damage in your body, therefore you can move naturally again. It's quite safe to move in a relaxed and graceful way.

You may get twinges of pain as you change from unnatural to natural movement. However, it's never as bad as you anticipate, and many people find (to their surprise) that they're able to do the movements they were avoiding at all costs with minimal discomfort. This is a major piece of getting out of pain, and I encourage you to explore it – starting today.

To see videos of these movements, go to www.6KeysPainFree.com and opt in for all the bonus material.

Natural Movement Examples

Transition from Lying to Sitting Up in Bed

In my clinic I often need people to lie down on the treatment bed so I can examine them. When they view the bed with extreme trepidation, I know this movement is something we'll need to explore. Getting out of bed involves two movements – rolling over and moving to a sitting position. We will look at both of these movements separately below and you can put them together.

Getting Out of Bed

This is something that killed me every morning for seven years. I used to get a ten of out ten shooting pain in my back and down my leg with the first movement. I started each morning in a cold sweat. However, there is another way. The most common thing people do to move their body from where they lie to the edge of the bed, is to tense their back and lift their pelvis in order to slide.

Instead, use your lower leg to gently push you along, and hook your arm over the side of the bed to pull you, so you can slide to the edge of the bed. You then bend your legs so they're hanging over the edge of the bed. Lever yourself up with your arms, using your legs as a counterweight. You do this in one movement with no twisting. If you use satin sheets, sliding is much easier.

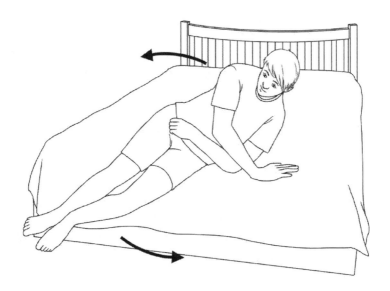

Rolling Over

In my clinic, I often need to ask someone lying on the examination bed to roll over, either from side to side or front to back. Sometimes, instead of rolling over, they get up, walk around to the other side of the bed, then lie down again – this time on their other side.

"Why did you do that?" I ask.

They look at me surprised. "Because it hurts my back to roll over and this is how I have solved the problem."

This is a very disruptive movement adaptation. It means you're going to wake every time you roll over (often waking your partner as well). The loss in sleep quality over time makes your pain system more sensitised, starting a downward spiral.

So here's how to roll over in a way that won't hurt. The underlying reason for pain when you roll is that you tense and lift your pelvis just prior to rolling over. You then twist your body. It is these movements that set off the pain.

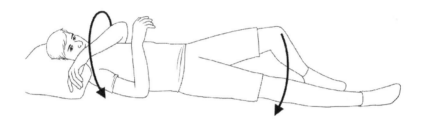

The secret is to see your body as a log with legs and arms attached. Your arms and legs become the levers to help roll the 'log' over, and you don't twist your spine.

If you are lying on your side, move your upper arm and leg backwards and roll onto your back. Then shift your other arm and leg over your body and roll like a log onto the other side. You can then slide into position; there is no need to lift your body. You do need more room for this, but it is infinitely better than heaving yourself up, groaning, moaning and waking yourself and your partner. As you practice this movement, it will rapidly become your default, and you'll be able to do this while asleep.

Transition from Sitting to Standing

This is what I see in my clinic: as a patient prepares to get out of the chair, they lean their whole body back. They breathe in, tense all their muscles, brace against the chair arms and very slowly lever themselves up, grimacing and wincing the whole time because it hurts.

This is a movement people do dozens of times a day. And if it hurts every time, this will really take the edge off life. The problem is, when people think it will hurt, the way they get out of a chair is guaranteed to produce more pain. If your weight is backwards as you get out of a chair, you're creating more pressure in your back, hips and knees. You're trying to avoid pain, but you're making it much worse.

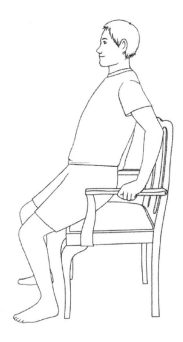

I get it. It's no fun having pain every time you get up. The problem is if you continue to get up in this way, your pain will continue to be just as bad.

Here's what you need to do: remember how you used to get out of a chair when you were a child? If you tried to do this and drew a blank, I'm not surprised. Most people do. This is because you never once thought about getting up when you were a kid. You were sitting down and thought 'I want to go there', and – voila! – you were up and out of the chair and heading in that direction. This is what you need to regain if you're going to get out of a chair with no pain.

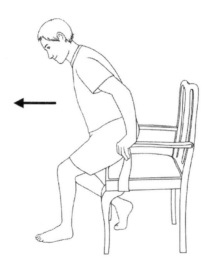

Here's what to do. When you're ready to stand, brace one foot backwards under the chair, and put one foot forwards as if you were going to take a step. You'll find that one foot naturally likes to be forward, the other backwards. For most people – if they're right handed – their left foot feels better forward, and vice versa.

Then, instead of leaning back in your chair and bracing your body with your arms, lean forward. Shift your bottom forward to the edge of the chair. Fix your gaze and your attention on where you want to go. This is also the time to start diaphragmatic breathing, letting your body know there is no threat here, and your muscles (and pain system) can relax.

If your chair has arms, you're allowed to give yourself a push off with your hands – for one second only. What you're *not* allowed to do is slowly heave yourself up, braced by your arms.

When your feet are in position, and your upper body is leaning forward, take a breath in, and as you breathe out, power off your back foot, lift your whole body forward and take a step in one fluid motion.

When I coach people through this in my clinic, I tell them, "You may feel a twinge as you get up, but instead of it lasting fifteen long seconds, it'll be for one moment and then you'll be moving and it'll be gone."

And, to people's great surprise and delight, this is exactly what happens. They're up and moving before their pain system has a chance to get the amplifiers dialled up. And as you get accustomed to this natural way of rising, you'll stop anticipating pain and the movement will become even more easy and comfortable.

I love seeing the astonishment in people's eyes as the movement they'd dreaded for years becomes something quite different – a long-lost friend from childhood they'd forgotten they knew.

Standing

Standing without pain means you can get out and about much easier. You'll be able to stand in queues in shops, wait for traffic lights on street corners, and start to resume your social life where you often stand talking at parties. The main issue with pain while standing is the way in which people approach it.

If you took one hundred soldiers and stood them in military posture (with both feet on a line parallel to their shoulders) for a couple of hours, at the end of that time, almost all of them would have sore backs. Unfortunately, most people think about standing in one of two ways – the stiff and upright 'correct' posture, and the inevitable slump when the muscles maintaining this posture become exhausted.

There is another way to stand, and you can learn this from looking at martial arts. It's universal. No martial art posture is completely front on, with both feet directly below your shoulders. This is because in this position, you can be easily pushed backwards.

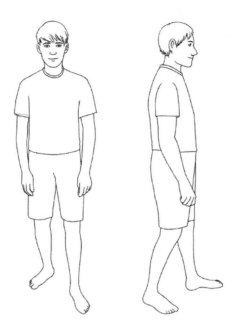

Most martial arts will have one foot slightly behind the other in what is called the 'lunge' position. This creates greater stability and range of motion in your body. It provides a better foundation for your spine, and gives you the option of transferring weight forward or backward to prevent fatigue in your lower legs. All in all, it's a much more efficient and comfortable way to stand.

Interestingly there is a 'primitive reflex' that all babies have before a year of age. If you posture them by moving one foot behind the other (one foot forward), the baby's spine is unchanged, but the other foot forward, the baby's spine straightens effortlessly. The foot that goes behind will usually be the same side as the dominant hand (though you will obviously only find this out later with each baby).

So instead of standing in the traditional way – with both feet squarely under your shoulders (meaning as you get tired), you'll shift weight between your legs and throw one hip out to compensate) – stand in a slight lunge. Put one foot slightly forward (you'll find one leg naturally feels better forward). When you do this, you turn on the same primitive reflex and your spine straightens effortlessly.

Practice taking this stance and rocking your hips forward and backward, transferring your weight between your legs. Feel the flexibility of movement and stability in this posture. Most people find they're able to stand for a longer time, and much more comfortably when they use this as a base.

Sitting

Sitting has been called 'the new smoking' because it's bad for our health in so many ways[3,4]. It's definitely a part of our modern chronic pain epidemic. We simply weren't designed to sit for the eight to ten hours a day that most office workers do.

To stay healthy, experts recommend you need to take a break and stand for one minute every thirty minutes[5]. This minimum dose gets blood flowing and muscles working, and was discovered by NASA scientists in their work with astronauts[6] They experimented with sedentary human beings on earth to simulate the extreme muscle and bone density loss astronauts were suffering in space.

Humans lying prone would suffer similar ill effects (not quite as fast as astronauts). Sitting for long periods causes the same problem – again not as dramatically – but quite measurably. But, if every thirty minutes you stand up for one minute, your body gets 'reset' and can maintain healthy muscle mass, bone density and circulation.

There's also better ways to sit than the usual office chair slump. The important thing to know with sitting is that your hip joint will only give you sixty degrees of flexion. This means for you to get your leg at a 90 degree to your back – as everyone does when they sit on a seat – the extra 30 degrees of bend has to come from somewhere. And that place is your spine.

Sitting normally destroys the natural curve of your spine (A) and puts pressure on your lower and upper back. Over time, this will often lead to back pain.

There are two options for healthier sitting. The first is to have a lumbar support behind your back. This is most commonly used, but it means your back is passively supported.

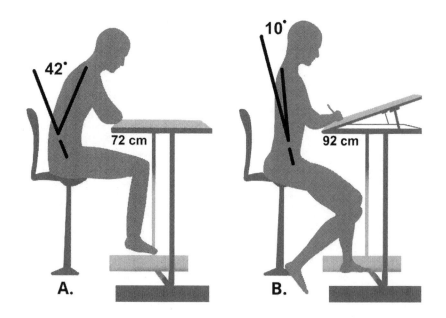

There is a better way to sit where your back stays active. Perch on the front end of your seat **(B)** so you can then tuck one leg under the chair. Another option is to tilt the seat itself forward or use a wedge cushion. This keeps the flexion of your hip at less than sixty degrees, and therefore your lower back can drop easily into its natural curve. This is seen in picture below. This is an active movement, therefore it strengthens your core and is more healthy in the long term. People who understand these principles can transition between both ways during the day. However, their back will be in optimum position all the time.

Lifting

The classic advice 'lift like a forklift not a crane' is still valid. So many people I see come to me after they lifted something heavy at an awkward angle – like a suitcase off an airport carousel. Something went 'ping' in their back and the pain began and never stopped.

Your disc has a thick wall (the annulus) with jelly in the middle (the nucleus pulposis). This acts as a shock absorber. If the spine is vertical and you put pressure onto the disc, the force will be distributed equally around the disc wall. The annulus is surprisingly strong and therefore, if you are strong enough to lift the weight, your disc should be able to cope. To lift safely, you need to keep your spine vertical. Like a weight lifter, you lift with the object straight in front of you, and keep it close to your body. This uses your major muscles – the biceps, quads, and gluteals.

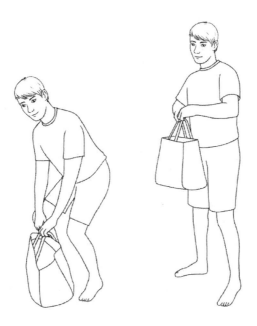

You can injure yourself when you start trying to lift things at odd angles while twisting and stretching outside your comfortable range. When you lean out and stretch to pick up an object, you increase the weight of the object because your arm becomes a lever and this magnifies the force. If you then twist at the same time, the force goes onto one corner of your disc, which may cause it to tear.

In normal life, this can happen when you are leaning into a car boot to lift out shopping, twisting to lift something off the back seat of your car, pulling a suitcase off an airport carousel etc. Under these conditions, pull the object towards you first, or step as close to the object as possible. Only then lift it close to your body, thereby allowing the forces to be spread evenly around the disc wall.

Turning Your Neck

I once talked to a lady who told me: "If I turn to my right more than thirty degrees, I hit the Wall of Pain." This Wall of Pain is fairly common for people with neck problems. Often it's when you turn just to one side (or it could be both sides). So people stop turning their head past the point where it hurts and this trims the edges of your vision, and your life. It also impacts on other activities, including safely driving your car.

The key to mobilising your neck is to see the movement you want – turning your head – as part of a larger pattern. Picture a larger spiral of movement – a whole kinetic chain – going up through your body. The end result is an effortless pain-free turning of your head.

If you want to turn to the right, the spiral starts right from the sole of your left foot. Shift your weight into the ball of this foot to begin the turn. Then, turn your hips slightly to your right. This spirals up through your spine and causes a slight turn in your back, shoulders, and finally your head. Turning your eyes to the right will further increase the range of movement and make it effortless.

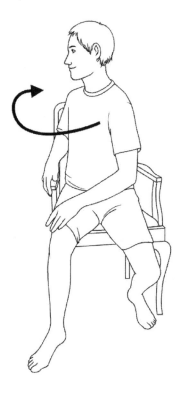

You achieve far greater movement this way, and not just because you're turning your whole body. What you've done is engage all the surrounding muscles, freeing up the facet joints in your neck and turning off the pain response you habitually have. Your whole body now dances as one.

I've seen people get fifteen to thirty degrees more turn in their neck within a few minutes. They're also able to do the movement pain free. The way to get past the Wall of Pain is not to try and blast away at it head on, that just makes it worse. When you include your neck turn as part of a larger spiral of movement, you effortlessly flow past the pain point and regain the lost mobility in your neck.

Shower Exercises

Every morning when I shower, I run through a series of exercises. They're in the bonus section at www.6KeysPainFree.com. You can do these exercises (or any others you like), but what I really recommend is the habit of doing some form of stretching every day. Doing stretches in the shower is great for two reasons: you have lovely hot water flowing over you, making your muscles relaxed and limber. Also, you have a shower each day at the same time, so it makes it much easier to embed this habit as a daily practice.

These are the common day-to-day movements many people need to relearn. However, you may have specific movement patterns you need to retrain. Next, we're going to explore mind and body tools you can use to regain pain-free movement.

Body Scanning and the Search for Comfort

We are hardwired to scan our body, searching for any areas that don't "feel right". This occurs without thought and is part of how we stay safe. When you have a normally-functioning pain system it's a useful habit.

However, when your pain system starts to malfunction, scanning your body and focusing on the pain message will feed the pain. Once you understand the pain you're feeling is coming from a malfunction, then it makes sense to do something different.

The problem is, it's very difficult (albeit impossible) to *not* scan your body. It's like trying to not think of a pink hippopotamus... you just did, right? However, you can replace 'scanning for pain' with 'scanning for comfort'.

As you become aware you're starting a body scan, focus your attention on the parts of your body that feel comfortable. If you have pain on one side, it's very useful to focus on the 'good' side instead. For example, if you have pain in your left hip, then focus your attention on the right hip. As you do, you can also speak to your sore hip and explain that this is how you want it to feel. You're using your mirror neurons to let the good side teach the bad side.

I saw Margaret a couple of years ago. She had had pain in her neck for years. As with many of my patients she had seen lots of experts and no one had been able to reduce her pain by any degree. When I saw her, I injected a small dose of local anaesthetic into the various trigger points around her neck and right shoulder, and explained there may be a small flare up of pain but that it would settle.

When I saw her ten days later she said that for the first time in many years her pain had gone completely. I was delighted, and said, "That's wonderful, what then happened?"

She said, "Well, what I did was, I searched for the pain that had disappeared. I kept searching for it continually and it took me three days to find the pain. And now it's back!"

She must have seen me with my jaw open and a look of shock on my face. "Why did you do that?" I asked.

I explained to her how her pain system works, and how to scan for comfort instead. The light of understanding came into her eyes. I repeated the treatment and told her because it had worked last time, it will definitely work this time. And it did.

After the shots, she focused only on the other side of her neck, which didn't hurt at all. I asked her to continually enjoy the feeling of movement without pain and to teach the right side that this is completely normal. And the good news is that after a few more injections, her pain never returned.

This story shows the incredible power of your mind to help or harm. If you assiduously look for your pain, you can and will find it. However, if you focus on areas of ease and comfort, your pain system will respond accordingly.

Mirror Neurons[7,8]

The reason using your good side to teach your bad side works is because of mirror neurons. These are special neurons in your brain that you use to copy movement. They are used socially (we see how people behave in a situation and model this) but they can also be used to learn new movements.

There's been some exciting research in the field of stroke recovery where people use their good side to help their stroke-afflicted side relearn how to move. You can do the same thing with pain if you have pain in one limb, or on one side of your body. I've taught this technique to people with pain in one leg, knee, arm, shoulder, hip, hand, and on one side of their back or neck.

Here's an example for people who have pain in one shoulder. People with shoulder pain usually adapt their movement to minimise their pain. To start using your mirror neurons, stand in front of a mirror. Put your opposite hand on your good shoulder, and slowly move your arm up and around. Feel how the muscles shift and dynamically adapt as you move your arm. As you raise your arm, feel how the whole shoulder drops slightly. Feel the sense of comfort and ease. Pay close attention to this, and store it in your memory.

Now, place the hand from your good side on your sore shoulder. To begin with, move it in the most comfortable and natural arc. For most people, this is the movement of bringing your hand up to your mouth.

While you are doing this, keep in your mind the image and the feeling of how your good shoulder moved. Tell your other shoulder this is how you would like it to move and feel as well. Keep within your range of comfortable movement at first. Then, slowly expand this range. However, don't force anything, and if you feel pain, retreat to the comfortable range again.

This is a great opportunity to practice diaphragmatic breathing (chapter 9). Deep, slow breathing sends a message to your pain system that you are not in danger, and it can relax. Practice this movement for a few minutes once or twice a day. The aim is to explore and re-examine what's possible for your body.

To their delight, many have found that the movements they've guarded against for so many years are not actually as painful as they once were. And, using their mirror neurons, they are able to relearn their natural pain-free way of moving.

Action Step #3

Finally, there's one more thing you need to get back to healthy, active movement. It's called an <u>Incremental Exercise Program.</u>

If you're in pain, getting active is difficult. For a start, moving hurts. And then, there's always the fear of flaring your pain when you exercise. However, you need to get active because exercise is a big part of breaking the pain cycle. When you exercise, your body produces endorphins – natural painkillers. And when you get a little bit conditioned, your muscles are stronger and less likely to get trigger points (chapter 10). Exercise is an important key to creating the virtuous cycle upwards and out of chronic pain.

To get people active again, I prescribe something called an incremental exercise program.
It's for those who have been so incapacitated by chronic pain, they've stopped exercising altogether. However, if you are able to exercise, the concept is still relevant.

In chapter 12 you saw how the pattern of boom and bust many people follow is prolonging and feeding the chronic pain cycle. If you stick to the method I'm about to describe when you exercise, you will do much better.

The incremental exercise program works like this: if you have been incredibly inactive for months because of your pain, the first step to do today is walk to your letterbox and back. That's it. Give yourself a pat on the back and know today's exercise is done. Repeat this for five to seven days.

Then walk out to your letterbox, turn right and walk to the first telephone pole or street light and back. That's all. If you don't have telephone poles on your street then walk about fifty yards. Repeat this for a few days. Then walk to the second telephone pole. Are you starting to see a pattern here? Every few days add just one telephone pole or fifty yards to your walk. The goal is getting you to the point of doing maximal aerobic exercise.

Aerobic exercise means that you can talk, whistle or sing while you're walking. It means your body is not being strained, but you are getting your heart rate up and getting moving. The magic moment comes when you are able to walk for half an hour comfortably. This is the point at which your body will reliably produce endorphins. Thirty minutes aerobic exercise per day means your body has started making its own natural painkillers. These are more powerful than morphine and have no side effects. Using energy during the day also means you're going to sleep better at night. And so the virtuous spiral upwards begins.

In the past I've given a prescription for people to get a puppy from a dog rescue shelter. When you have a supremely excitable puppy begging you to go outside, disciplining yourself to take your daily walk is out of your hands. And as the puppy grows and needs to walk longer distances, you'll also be able to walk further.

I recommend doing this slowly-increasing walk six days out of seven. While you're doing your walk, tell yourself it is going to be amazingly good for you. Because it is. Tell your body how it's now going to produce endorphins to naturally turn down your pain and give you ease of movement.

Here's a story to illustrate why you should do this. A group of maids[9] working in a hotel were asked by researchers how much exercise they did. They all replied "Not much." Next, half of them were shown how, due to their cleaning work, which involved lifting, pushing, carrying and bending, they actually did more exercise than the Surgeon General recommended per day. The other maids weren't told anything.

Several weeks later, the researchers measured the weight loss of all the maids. They discovered something interesting. The ones who had been told their daily work was excellent exercise, had lost weight and were in physically better condition. They weren't doing any extra exercise. Only their understanding had changed. The maids who hadn't been told anything were in exactly the same condition.

Your brain is the most powerful organ in your body. So when you exercise, remind yourself how this is fundamentally changing your health and starting a positive spiral in your daily life.

With just a small amount of regular exercise you will return to comfortable movement and a rich quality of life. Each day gradually increase till you reach the magic thirty minutes a day of gentle aerobic exercise. And as you do this you will notice how profoundly this adds to your feeling of well-being and health.

14

Life After Pain

We've covered a lot of ground so far. Like any journey, there will be roadblocks that set you back. We're going to go through some of these now.

Some people start doing their mind-body, breathing, and movement practice, and as soon as they notice some improvement they lose focus and stop. Everything grinds to a halt, and it's only when their pain starts to intrude on their life that they begin again. Their progress looks like the graph below:

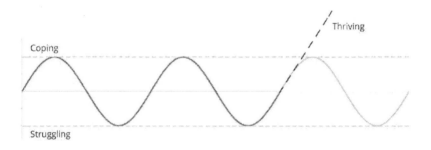

When you are starting to have success with a technique, the key is to KEEP GOING! You will get busy, and life will intervene. However, the people who are consistent make the most dramatic progress.

A wonderful way to be consistent, and track your daily habits is to keep a journal. This makes you accountable to yourself, and keeps you focused on your long-term goals.

Another huge help is to join a group of like-minded people who are walking the same walk. You can find a group like this on www.LifeAfterPain.com, and join.

Another roadblock people encounter is the perfectly normal human desire to keep gathering information. Information is interesting and satisfies your curiosity, but it is no substitute for actually doing the work. I sometimes meet people in my online community who are stuck in this mode. They ask lots of intelligent questions, but when I ask them what they've put into practice, the answer is: not much.

This is not a theoretical topic. Like swimming, you can't learn it just by reading and understanding it. You need to do it! As the ancient philosopher Lao Tzu said: "A journey of a thousand miles begins with a single step."

Take that step. While knowledge is empowering, you will learn more in your first ten minutes of mind-body practice than you will by reading one hundred books.

The next roadblock is discouragement due to pain flares. In your journey towards a pain-free life, there will be ups and downs. In fact, it's expected. Think about it logically; your pain system has set up this amplified pain in a mistaken attempt to protect you. When you start challenging it, this sometimes sets off a pain flare. It's a last ditch attempt by your pain system to maintain the status quo and keep you 'safe'.

When you have a setback, the temptation is to think you have not made any progress and are back where you started. The key here is to batten down, and keep on keeping on. (Or as Winston Churchill put it: "When you are going through hell, keep going.")

I find it helpful to see your journey as progress toward a distant mountain peak. You will need to cross valleys and plateaus to get there. Sometimes it will feel like you're going backwards. But as long as you put one foot in front of the other, you will get there in the end.

It also helps to change your focus. When you feel like you're not progressing, look back and see how far you've come. If you're always looking at how far you have to go, your experience will be one of continual dissatisfaction and struggle. If instead you take regular checks on your small wins and celebrate your victories, your experience will be one of encouragement. Again, this is where a daily journal recording your practice is useful.

A final helper is to put your attention on getting back to doing the things you love rather than being pain free. Being pain free will come, but it will come slower if your main focus is on your pain. Make doing the work your daily target, rather than the results. Concentrate on doing the practices, breathing freely and mindfully enjoying activities that previously you'd avoided. This removes pain as the central focus of your life, and makes the whole journey more rewarding.

Jill had painful feet whenever she walked more than thirty minutes. So instead of trying to walk for longer without pain (thus putting all her attention on her feet to see if they were painful), she tried walking barefoot on soft grass.

Her attention was taken up with the pleasurable sensation of the grass on her bare feet. She told me it had never occurred to her in years that she could rediscover the pleasures of walking. And as she made this a habit, her pain diminished.

Whenever possible, look for opportunities to experience bliss, comfort, and joy in 'everyday' things. Now you know what causes your pain – and that it isn't dangerous – you can stop worrying and thinking about it. Remember, the key problem is in your pain system. It is there to keep you safe, but it has become confused about what that means and is sending you amplified pain messages. As you retrain it, it will turn the pain messages down, and you will observe your pain lessening day by day.

The truth is that our bodies are incredible at healing. Given time, they will heal almost any injury, and they can and will heal it to the stage where you can use your body without pain.

The Magic Moment

I want to take some time to describe a particular moment for you, because I'm worried that if I don't, it will slip by without you noticing. Like it did for me.

This comes after you have been practising a mind-body technique for some days or weeks. The magic moment is, you feel the pain, and as a reflex you apply your technique and the pain lessens.

What has happened is that your pain system has sent you an amplified pain message, and without conscious thought, your mind-body technique has stopped the process in its tracks. In this moment, you've reversed what went wrong in the first place to cause your chronic pain. You have retrained your pain system to behave normally – like it used to.

In technical terms, you've engaged – automatically – your descending inhibitory pathway. You have mobilised your command centre (your brain), which has then up-regulated soothing neurotransmitters in your spinal cord. These then turn down your pain.

When you experience this personally, it's like your pain tried to start growing, and then you stepped in and said "NO!"

"No, I don't have time for this spam pain message. It's not useful or helpful, and so I'm going to delete it."

It is truly a magic moment. And as I said before, mine slipped by without me even registering it. I just noticed my pain was hardly bothering me. I was getting back into doing my beloved sports, and not having to pay for them later with low back pain and sciatica.

It was truly like being reborn. I was again becoming the engaged, happy, and active person I had previously been. Except this time, I didn't take it for granted. And I still practice gratitude to this day.

This is what I want you to experience. It is completely possible. Because for people in chronic pain, most – and sometimes all of their pain – is being caused by a malfunction in their pain system.

This process takes practice, experimentation, and dedication. But with the right keys you can and will return your pain system to normal. I have coached numerous people through this process.

Now, it's your turn.

It's time to take the Six Keys and unlock your pain-free life. Here's a recap of what you've learned:

1. The First Key is the understanding of what is causing your pain. In particular, the three pain types and how they create pain long after your body has healed. Once you have this understanding, you then work out which pain type you are.

2. The Second Key is to develop your daily mind-body practice to reset your pain system. You may need to try two to three mind-body techniques till you find the one that resonates with you. Once you have, practice this mind-body technique day and night, every time you feel pain, until it becomes part of you. In other words, you make it a habit.

3. The Third Key is diaphragmatic breathing. Combine breathing with your chosen mind-body technique. This will enhance its power and further turn down your autonomic and pain system. Do this until breathing and your mind-body practice are inseparable. The Fourth Key: learn how to treat triggers points, and combine this treatment with breathing. Use your judgement to decide how much of the trigger treatment you need. If the mind-body technique is going really well, then do less. However, if you're struggling to get dramatic improvement through mind-body techniques,

then trigger treatment gives you a good entry point into this world.

4. Key Five: once your mind-body technique is a solid daily practice running on auto-pilot, it's time to go deeper. Review your unconscious and the hidden emotional drivers of pain. Through this exploration, start noticing and questioning your beliefs and repetitive thought patterns. Apply breathing and the mind-body techniques you already know to interrupt these repetitive loops throughout your day.

5. The final Sixth Key is natural movement. By this stage, you will be adept at breathing and your mind-body practice. You can therefore do these as you change your movement patterns. This will make the transition back to natural movement faster, and will link it more effectively to your pain system reset.

What you're doing is adding layers. The secret is to make each key habitual, and then integrate the next key into it. When you combine all the techniques, they create a whole that is more powerful than the sum of its parts. Your pain system – mind and body – has no choice but to return to its natural, normal state.

This all leads to your life after pain.

15

Moving Forward (and the Meaning of Life)

"Before enlightenment, chop wood and carry water. After enlightenment, chop wood and carry water." ~ Zen Saying

The meaning of life is a fairly ambitious topic to address… but why not! After all, we've come this far together.

I want to prepare you for re-entering a pain-free life because I have confidence that as you master these techniques, this will be your future. So here are a few observations I think you will find useful as you make this transition.

Many people in chronic pain remember a rose-tinted past before their pain began. And it's partially true. Chronic pain makes everything harder. It takes the edge off life and sucks the joy out of it. But your life before you had pain was not perfect. Remembering it like this will only sharpen your suffering now.

As pain is successfully turned down, some people enter a stage of grieving. They mourn the time they lost while they were in pain. There's nothing wrong with this, and it can be healthy to grieve as long as you then move on. Remembering that your life before you had pain wasn't perfect may help you move out of this mourning phase sooner (if you do enter into it).

Remember, there is no perfect 'there'. No happily ever after. Conquering this one challenge means you move on to other challenges. However, you will have grown in the process.

You will be a different person than you were. You will have gained hard-earned knowledge from your journey through the valley of pain. I want to make sure you take this knowledge with you because it has been won by the bitterest struggle and sacrifice.

You can bring this wisdom into other parts of your life. I encourage you to share it with those around you to enrich their lives and yours. You will be stronger and more compassionate than before.

When you have safely moved out of the chronic pain cycle, and back to normal life, you may find you need to rediscover your purpose. How to do that is outside the scope of this book. However, I offer you this:

The world needs people like you, those who have looked deep within themselves, and gathered their courage, hope and determination to overcome obstacles others cannot even imagine. Whatever you decide to make of your life after pain, know that it will be worth it. You will create something unique with your life – something only you can do.

I look forward to meeting you one day, and thank you for sharing your life with those of us who are still in the trenches, doing what we can each day to live well. We need what only you have to offer.

Go do it.

Acknowledgements

We'd like to thank the readers of LifeAfterPain.com for their support. Eira Kuttner for being the rock. The Book Club members for their insightful comments. Amanda Spedding for her wonderful editing, clarity and help. And the many kind and generous people who helped us share this book with their audiences. Yoav Ezer, for his wise guidance. My patients who, over the years, have taught me more than any medical institution. My son Benjamin, for being our most honest critic. My sister Dr Leora Kuttner, for wisdom and encouragement. And the pioneers and researchers of chronic pain medicine, whose ongoing work continues to help people get their lives back from chronic pain.

Download the '6 Keys Pain Free' Bonus Package

Which includes:

- A video guide to understanding amplified pain
- The Trigger Point Finder Tool: to help you effortlessly find triggers anywhere in your body for fast pain relief
- Video guide on how to most effectively find and treat trigger points
- Natural movement examples for pain-free movement
- The 3 Chronic Pain Types Quiz – find out which pain type you are
- A guided audio recording on breathing for stress and pain relief
- Simple exercises you can do each morning to regain core strength
- And much more....

To download your Free Bonus Package click the link below (if you are using a digital reader) or type this URL into your browser...

www.6KeysPainFree.com

A call to post a review

Helping thousands of people with chronic pain has taught me a lot about treating chronic pain. And I've done my best to share the techniques and strategies I've learned with you in this book.

But I'm just learning my way as an author.

That's why I need your help...

It would be immensely helpful to me if you could write a review for this book and publish it on Amazon.

To write the review, go to my book page on amazon:

www.StayPainFree.com (this url will redirect you to Amazon) Scroll down to the reviews section.

And just write an honest review (good or bad) and give my book as many stars as you think it deserves.

Thank you in advance,
Dr Jonathan Kuttner

About the Authors:

Dr Jonathan Kuttner (MBBCH, Dip Sports Med, Dip MSM, FRNZCGP, FAFMM) is a musculo-skeletal pain specialist who has spent the last 35 years working as a doctor in New Zealand. He is the recipient of the NAMTPT Lifetime Award for Contribution to Myofascial Trigger Point Therapy and has been featured on national TV and radio in Australia and New Zealand.

Naomi Kuttner partnered with her father Jonathan to write this book. She is an online business and publishing specialist.

Further Reading

The Mindbody Prescription – Dr John Sarno

The Trigger Point Therapy Workbook Book – Clair Davies & Amber Davies

The Power of Habit – Charles Duhigg

Wherever You Go, There You Are – Jon Kabat-Zinn

Foundation: Redefine Your Core, Conquer Back Pain, and Move with Confidence – Eric Goodman

The Fear and Anxiety Solution - Friedemann Schaub MD

References

Chapter 1

1. Mirza SK, Deyo RA. Systematic review of randomized trials comparing lumbar fusion surgery to non-operative care for treatment of chronic back pain. Spine. 2007;32:816–23.   doi: 10.1097/01.brs.0000259225.37454.38.

2. Slipman CW, Shin CH, Patel RK, et al. (Sep 2002). "Etiologies of failed back surgery syndrome". Pain Med. 3 (3):   200–14;   discussion   214–7. doi:10.1046/j.1526-4637.2002.02033.x. PMID 15099254

3. Fager C. A.; Freiberg S. R. (1980). "Analysis of failures and poor results of lumbar spine surgery." Spine. 5 (1): 87–94. doi:10.1097/00007632-198001000-00015

Chapter 2

1. Woolf C. Central sensitization: Implications for the diagnosis and treatment of pain. PAIN Volume 152, Issue 3, Supplement, March 2011, Pages S2–S15 Biennial Review of Pain.

2. Staud R, Vierck C et al. Abnormal sensitization and temporal summation of second pain (wind-up) in patients with fibromyalgia syndrome. PAIN Volume 91 Issues 1-2, March 2001, Pages 175-205

3. Woolf C, Salter M. Neuronal Plasticity: Increasing the Gain in Pain. Science 09 Jun 2000: Vol. 288, Issue 5472, pp. 1765-1768 DOI: 10.1126/science.288.5472.1765

4. Meeus M., & Nijs, J. (2007). Central sensitization: A biopsychosocial explanation for chronic widespread pain in patients with fibromyalgia and chronic fatigue syndrome. Clinical Journal of Rheumatology, 26, 465-473.

5. Verne, V. N., & Price, D. D. (2002). Irritable bowel syndrome as a common precipitant of central sensitization. Current Rheumatology Reports, 4, 322-328

6. Bajaj, P., Bajaj, P., Madsen, H., & Arendt-Nielsen, L. (2003). Endometriosis is associated with central sensitization: A psychophysical controlled study. The Journal of Pain, 4, 372-380

7. Coppola, G., DiLorenzo, C., Schoenen, J. & Peirelli, F. (2013). Habituation and sensitization in primary headaches. Journal of Headache and Pain, 14, 65

8. Melzack, R., Coderre, T. J., Kat, J., & Vaccarino, A. L. (2001). Central neuroplasticity and pathological pain. Annals of the New York Academy of Sciences, 933, 157-174.

9. Yunus, M. B. (2007). The role of central sensitization in symptoms beyond muscle pain, and the evaluation of a patient with widespread pain. Best Practice Research in Clinical Rheumatology, 21, 481-497

10. Curatolo, M., Arendt-Nielsen, L., & Petersen-Felix, S. (2006). Central hypersensitivity in chronic pain: Mechanisms and clinical implications. Physical Medicine and Rehabilitation Clinics of North America, 17, 287-302.

11. O'Neill, S., Manniche, C., Graven-Nielsen, T., Arendt-Nielsen, L. (2007). Generalized deep-tissue

hyperalgesia in patients with chronic low-back pain. European Journal of Pain, 11, 415-420.

12. Banic, B, Petersen-Felix, S., Andersen O. K., Radanov, B. P., Villiger, P. M., Arendt-Nielsen, L., & Curatolo, M. (2004). Evidence for spinal cord hypersensitivity in chronic pain after whiplash injury and fibromyalgia. Pain, 107, 7-15

13. Meeus M., Vervisch, S., De Clerck, L. S., Moorkens, G., Hans, G., & Nijs, J. (2012). Central sensitization in patients with rheumatoid arthritis: A systematic literature review. Seminars in Arthritis & Rheumatism, 41, 556-567

14. Fernandez-Lao, Cantarero-Villanueva, I., Fernandez-de-Las-Penas, C, Del-Moral-Avila, R., Arendt-Nielsen, L., Arroyo-Morales, M. (2010). Myofascial trigger points in neck and shoulder muscles and widespread pressure pain hypersensitivity in patients with post-mastectomy pain: Evidence of peripheral and central sensitization. Clinical Journal of Pain, 26, 798-806.

Chapter 3

1. Hassed C, Mind-body therapies–use in chronic pain management. Aust Fam Physician. 2013 Mar;42(3):112-7.

2. Lee C, Crawford C, Hickey A. Mind-body therapies for the self-management of chronic pain symptoms. Pain Med. 2014 Apr;15 Suppl 1:S21-39. doi: 10.1111/pme.12383.

3. Astin JA. Mind-body therapies for the management of pain. Clin J Pain. 2004 Jan-Feb;20(1):27-32.

4. Saarto T, Wiffen PJ. Antidepressants for neuropathic pain. Cochrane Database Syst Rev. 2007;4:CD005454.

5. Dworkin RH, O'Connor AB, Backonja M, et al. Pharmacologic management of neuropathic pain: evidence-based recommendations. Pain. 2007;132:237-251.

6. Sawynok J, Esser M, Reid A. Antidepressants as analgesics: an overview of central and peripheral mechanisms of action. J Psychiatry Neurosci. 2001 Jan; 26(1): 21–29

7. Blier P, Abbott FV. Putative mechanisms of action of antidepressant drugs in affective and anxiety disorders and pain. J Psychiatry Neurosci. 2001;26:37-43.

8. Brannan SK, Mallinckrodt CH, Brown EB, et al. Duloxetine 60 mg once-daily in the treatment of painful physical symptoms in patients with major depressive disorder. J Psychiatr Res. 2005;39:43-53.

9. Bradley RH, Barkin RL, Jerome J, et al. Efficacy of venlafaxine for the long term treatment of chronic pain with associated major depressive disorder. Am J Ther. 2003;10:318-323.

Chapter 4

1. Mackintosh, N. J. (1983). Conditioning and associative learning (p. 316). Oxford: Clarendon Press.

2. Pavlov, I. P., & Anrep, G. V. (2003). Conditioned reflexes. Courier Corporation.

3. Watson, J. B. (2013). Behaviorism. Read Books Ltd.

4. Woolf C, Salter M. Neuronal Plasticity: Increasing the Gain in Pain. Science 09 Jun 2000: Vol. 288, Issue 5472, pp. 1765-1768 DOI: 10.1126/science.288.5472.1765

5. Murakami M, Hirano T. The molecular mechanisms of chronic inflammation development. Front Immunol.

2012; 3: 323. Published online 2012 Nov 15. doi:10.3389/fimmu.2012.00323

6. Cheung K, Hume P, Maxwell L. Delayed Onset Muscle Soreness Treatment Strategies and Performance Factors. Sports Med 2003; 33 (2): 145-16

7. Schogren P, Fisher R et al Stand up for health – avoiding sedentary behaviour might lengthen your telomeres: secondary outcomes from a physical activity RCT in older people. Br J Sports Med doi:10.1136/bjsports-2013-093342.

8. Hassed C, Mind-body therapies–use in chronic pain management. Aust Fam Physician. 2013 Mar;42(3):112-7.

9. Lee C, Crawford C, Hickey A. Mind-body therapies for the self-management of chronic pain symptoms. Pain Med. 2014 Apr;15 Suppl 1:S21-39. doi: 10.1111/pme.12383.

10. Astin JA. Mind-body therapies for the management of pain. Clin J Pain. 2004 Jan-Feb;20(1):27-32.

11. Gallego, J., Nsegbe, E. and Durand, E. (2001). Learning in respiratory control. Behavior Modification, 25 (4) 495-512.

12. Pal, G.K. Velkumary, S. and Madanmohan. (2004). Effect of short-term practice of breathing exercises on autonomic functions in normal human volunteers. Indian Journal of Medical Research, 120, 115-121.

13. Sovik, R. (2000). The science of breathing – The yogic view. Progress in Brain Research, 122 (Chapter 34), 491-505.

Chapter 5

1. McCorry L. Physiology of the Autonomic Nervous System. Am J Pharm Educ. 2007 Aug 15; 71(4): 78

2. Adrenaline, Cortisol, Norepinephrine: The Three Major Stress Hormones, Explained. Hufflington Post. April 19, 2014. Retrieved 16 August 2014.

3. Jansen, A; Nguyen, X; Karpitsky, V; Mettenleiter, M. Central Command Neurons of the Sympathetic Nervous System: Basis of the Fight-or-Flight Response". Science Magazine. 27 October 1995.5236 270.

4. Olpin, Michael. "The Science of Stress". Weber State University

5. Ida J. Llewellyn-Smith and Anthony J. M. Verberne. Central Regulation of Autonomic Functions. Print publication date: 2011. Print ISBN-13: 9780195306637. Published to Oxford Scholarship Online: May 2011.

6. Manabe N1, Tanaka T, Hata J, Kusunoki H, Haruma K. Pathophysiology underlying irritable bowel syndrome–from the viewpoint of dysfunction of autonomic nervous system activity. J Smooth Muscle Res. 2009 Feb;45(1):15-23.

7. Hubeaux K1, Deffieux X, Raibaut P, Le Breton F, Jousse M, Amarenco G. Evidence for autonomic nervous system dysfunction in females with idiopathic overactive bladder syndrome. Neurourol Urodyn. 2011 Nov;30(8):1467-72. doi: 10.1002/nau.21154. Epub 2011 Jun 29.

8. Pal, G.K. Velkumary, S. and Madanmohan. (2004). Effect of short-term practice of breathing exercises on autonomic functions in normal human volunteers. Indian Journal of Medical Research, 120, 115-121.

9. Etienne Vachon-Presseau, Mathieu Roy, Marc-Olivier Martel, Etienne Caron, Marie-France Marin, Jeni Chen, Geneviève Albouy, Isabelle Plante, Michael J. Sullivan,

Sonia J. Lupien, Pierre Rainville. The stress model of chronic pain: evidence from basal cortisol and hippocampal structure and function in humans. DOI: http://dx.doi.org/10.1093/brain/aws371 815-827 First published online: 24 February 2013

10. Phillip J Quartana, PhD, Claudia M Campbell, PhD, and Robert R Edwards, PhD. Pain catastrophizing: a critical review. Expert Rev Neurother. 2009 May; 9(5): 745–758. doi: 10.1586/ERN.09.34

Chapter 6

1. Darrell J. Gaskin, Ph.D. and Patrick Richard, Ph.D., M.A. The Economic Costs of Pain in the United States. Relieving Pain in America: A Blueprint for Transforming Prevention, Care, Education, and Research.

2. David L. Sackett. Evidence-based medicine. Seminars in Perinatology Volume 21, Issue 1, February 1997, Pages 3-5

3. Evidence-Based Medicine Working Group (November 1992). "Evidence-based medicine. A new approach to teaching the practice of medicine". JAMA. 268 (17): 2420–5. doi:10.1001/jama.268.17.2420. PMID 1404801.

4. Donald D. Price,1 Damien G. Finniss,2 and Fabrizio Benedetti. A Comprehensive Review of the Placebo Effect: Recent Advances and Current Thought. Annual Review of Psychology Vol. 59: 565-590 (Volume publication date January 2008)

5. National Cancer Institute (n.d.). "NCI Dictionary of Cancer Terms: Levels of evidence". US DHHS-National Institutes of Health. Retrieved 8 December 2014.

6. Beck, A. The past and the future of cognitive therapy. Journal of Psychotherapy Practice and Research, 199) 6, 276-284.

7. Stewart B. Epidemiology of Chronic Pain. Geisinger
   . Centre for Health Research.

8. Hiroshi Minagawa,a Nobuyuki Yamamoto,b Hidekazu Abe,c Masashi Fukuda,d Nobutoshi Seki,c Kazuma Kikuchi,Chiroaki Kijima,c and Eiji Itoi. Prevalence of symptomatic and asymptomatic rotator cuff tears in the general population: From mass-screening in one village. J Orthop. 2013 Mar; 10(1): 8–12. Published online 2013 Feb 26. doi: 10.1016/j.jor.2013.01.008

9. Tempelhof S., Rupp S., Seil R. Age-related prevalence of rotator cuff tears in asymptomatic shoulders. J Shoulder Elbow Surg. 1999;8:296–299.

10. Kalichman L, Li L, Kim DH, Guermazi A, Berkin V, O'Donnell CJ, Hoffmann U, Cole R, Hunter DJ. Spondylolysis and spondylolisthesis: prevalence and association with low back pain in the adult community-based population. Spine (Phila Pa 1976). 2009 Jan 15; 34(2): 199–205. doi: 10.1097/BRS.0b013e31818edcfd

11. Andersson, G B. What are the age-related changes in the spine? Baillieres Clinical Rheumatology. 1998. 12(1):161-73, 1998 Feb.

12. van Tulder, M W. Assendelft, W J. Koes, B W. Bouter, L M.. Spinal radiographic findings and nonspecific low back pain. A systematic review of observational studies. Spine. 1997, 22(4):427-34, 1997 Feb 15.

Chapter 7

1. Edwards RR, Ness TJ, Weigent DA, Fillingim RB (December 2003). "Individual differences in diffuse noxious inhibitory controls (DNIC): association with clinical variables". Pain 106 (3): 427–37.

2. Baliki MN, Chialvo DR, Geha PY, Levy RM, Harden RN, Parrish TB, Apkarian AV. Chronic pain and the emotional brain: specific brain activity associated with spontaneous fluctuations of intensity of chronic back pain. J Neurosci. 2006;26:12165–12173.

3. Apkarian AV. Pain perception in relation to emotional learning. Curr Opin Neurobiol. 2008;18:464–468

Chapter 8

1. Ann M. Graybiel, The Basal Ganglia and Chunking of Action Repertoires, NEUROBIOLOGY OF LEARNING AND MEMORY 70, 119–136 (1998), ARTICLE NO. NL983843

2. A Vania Apkarian, The brain in chronic pain: clinical implications, Pain Manag. 2011 Nov 1; 1(6): 577–586.

Chapter 9

1. Hornsveld H, Garssen B, Dop MF, van Spiegel P. Symptom reporting during voluntary hyperventilation and mental load: implications for diagnosing hyperventilation syndrome. J Psychosom Res. 1990;34(6):687–697.

2. G Magarian. Hyperventilation Syndrome: Infrequently recognised common expressions of anxiety and stress. Medicine, vol. 64 no.12, 1989.

3. W N Gardner. The Pathophysiology of Hyperventilation Disorders. Chest, 109, Feb 1996.

4. Jones M, Harvey A, Marston L, O'Connell NE. Breathing exercises for dysfunctional breathing/hyperventilation syndrome in adults. Cochrane Database Syst Rev. 2013 May 31. 5:CD009041.

5. Bradley D. Hyperventilation Syndrome. Kyle Cathie Ltd. ISBN 9781856267502

Chapter 10

1. Travell, Janet; Simons David; Simons Lois (1999). Myofascial Pain and Dysfunction: The Trigger Point Manual (2 vol. set, 2nd Ed.). USA: Lippincott Williams & Williams. ISBN 9780683083637.

2. Simons DG . "New views of myofascial trigger points: etiology and diagnosis". Archives of Physical Medicine and Rehabilitation. 2008 89(1): 157–9. doi:10.1016/j.apmr.2007.11.016. PMID 18164347

3. Fernández-de-las-Peñas C, Cuadrado ML, Arendt-Nielsen L, Simons DG, Pareja JA. Myofascial trigger points and sensitization: an updated pain model for tension-type headache. Cephalalgia. doi:10.1111/j.1468-2982.2007.01295.

4. Fernandez-Lao, Cantarero-Villanueva, I., Fernandez-de-Las-Penas, C, Del-Moral-Avila, R., Arendt-Nielsen, L., Arroyo-Morales, M. (2010). Myofascial trigger points in neck and shoulder muscles and widespread pressure pain hypersensitivity in patients with post-mastectomy pain: Evidence of peripheral and central sensitization. Clinical Journal of Pain, 26, 798-806.

5. Myburgh, C; Larsen AH; Hartvigsen J. . "A systematic, critical review of manual palpation for identifying myofascial trigger points: evidence and clinical significance". Arch Phys Med Rehabil. 2008 89 (6):

1169–76.   doi:10.1016/j.apmr.2007.12.033.   PMID 18503816. Retrieved 2012-07-23.

6. Chen Q, Bensamoun S, Basford JR, Thompson JM, An KN . "Identification and quantification of myofascial taut bands with magnetic resonance elastography" (PDF). Archives of Physical Medicine and Rehabilitation. December 2007 88 (12): 1658–61. doi:10.1016/j.apmr.2007.07.020. PMID 18047882

7. Sharman, M., Cresswell, A. and Riek, S. Proprioceptive Neuromuscular Facilitation Stretching. Journal of Sports Medicine, 2006 36, 929-939

8. Melzack R, Stillwell DM, Fox EJ . "Trigger points and acupuncture points for pain: correlations and implications" (PDF). Pain. February 1977 3 (1): 3–23. doi:10.1016/0304-3959(77)90032-X. PMID 69288

9. "Trigger point injection". Non-Surgical Orthopaedic & Spine Center. October 2006. Archived from the original on 2006-10-26. Retrieved 2007-04-07.

Chapter 11

1. Woolf C. Central sensitization: Implications for the diagnosis and treatment of pain. PAIN Volume 152, Issue 3, Supplement, March 2011, Pages S2–S15 Biennial Review of Pain.

2. Gudin J. (2004). Medscape Neurobiology: Expanding Our Understanding of Central Sensitization. Medscape: Medscape Education.

3. Phillips, K. & Clauw, D. J. (2011). Central pain mechanisms in chronic pain states – maybe it is all in their head. Best Practice Research in Clinical Rheumatology, 25, 141-154.

4. Porta, M, ed. . "Natural history of disease". A Dictionary of Epidemiology (5th ed.).2014 Oxford: Oxford University Press. pp. 193–194. ISBN 978-0-19-939005-2

5. Borenstein DG, O'Mara JW Jr, Boden SD, et al. The value of magnetic resonance imaging of the lumbar spine to predict low-back pain in asymptomatic subjects. J Bone Joint Surg Am 2001;83-A:1306–1311.

6. Jordon J, Konstantinou K, O'Dowd J. Herniated lumbar disc. BMJ Clin Evid. v.2009;2009 PMC2907819

7. DePalma MJ, Bhargava A, Slipman CW. A critical appraisal of the evidence for selective nerve root injection in the treatment of lumbosacral radiculopathy. Arch Phys Med Rehabil 2005;86:1477–1483. Search date 2003; Primary sources Medline, Pubmed, Ovid, MDConsult, Embase, The Cochrane Library, and references lists.

8. Gibson JNA, Waddell G. Surgical interventions for lumbar disc prolapse. In: The Cochrane Library, Issue 2, 2008. Chichester, UK: John Wiley & Sons Ltd. Search date 2007

9. Jacobs WC, van Tulder M, Arts M, et al; Surgery versus conservative management of sciatica due to a lumbar herniated Eur Spine J. 2011 Apr;20(4):513-22. Epub 2010 Oct 15.

10. Mohamed M. Mohi Eldin1 and Naglaa M. Abdel Razek. Epidural Fibrosis after Lumbar Disc Surgery: Prevention and Outcome Evaluation. Asian Spine J. v.9(3); 2015 Jun PMC4472585

11. Nalini Sehgal, MD*, Joseph D. Fortin, DO. Internal Disc Disruption and Low Back Pain. Pain Physician,

Volume 3, Number 2, pp 143-157 2000, Association of Pain Management Anesthesiologists

12. Anderson P. Intervertebral Disc Arthroplasty. Spine 2004;29(23):2779-2786

13. Martin Krismer. Review article FUSION OF THE LUMBAR SPINE A consideration of the indications. European Instructional Course Lectures Vol. 5, 2001

14. Chou R, et al. (2009). Interventional therapies, surgery and interdisciplinary rehabilitation for low back pain: An evidence-based clinical practice guideline from the American Pain Society. Spine, 34(10): 1066-1077.

15. Leonid Kalichman and David J. Hunter Diagnosis and conservative management of degenerative lumbar spondylolisthesis. Eur Spine J v.17(3); 2008 Mar PMC2270383

16. JP Kostuik et al. The Incidence of Low-Back Pain in Adult Scoliosis. Spine (Phila Pa 1976) 6 (3), 268-273. May-Jun 1981.

17. Joseph A Janicki, MD1 and Benjamin Alman. Scoliosis: Review of diagnosis and treatment. Paediatr Child Health. 2007 Nov; 12(9): 771–776

18. Murphy L, Helmick CG.The impact of osteoarthritis in the United States: a population-health perspective. Am J Nurs. 2012;112(3 Suppl 1):S13-9

19. Adam P. Goode, PT, DPT, PhD,1, Timothy S. Carey, MD, MPH,2 and Joanne M. Jordan. Low Back Pain and Lumbar Spine Osteoarthritis: How Are They Related? Curr Rheumatol Rep. 2013 Feb; 15(2): 305. doi: 10.1007/s11926-012-0305-z

20. Laxmaiah Manchikanti et al. An Update of Comprehensive Evidence-Based Guidelines for Interventional Techniques in Chronic Spinal Pain. Part

II: Guidance and Recommendations. Pain Physician 2013; 16:S49-S283 • ISSN 1533-3159

21. Rush University Medical Center. "Cementless Hip Implants Are Durable For At Least 20 Years." ScienceDaily. ScienceDaily, 3 May 2009.

22. Malchau H, Herberts P. Prognosis of total hip replacement. The Swedish National Hip Arthroplasty register 1996. Proceedings American Academy of Orthopedic Surgeons. Atlanta: 1996.

23. American Academy of Orthopaedic Surgeons. "98 percent of total knee replacement patients return to life, work following surgery." ScienceDaily. ScienceDaily, 21 March 2013.

24. Chou R1, Baisden J, Carragee EJ, Resnick DK, Shaffer WO, Loeser JD. Surgery for low back pain: a review of the evidence for an American Pain Society Clinical Practice Guideline. Spine (Phila Pa 1976). 2009 May 1;34(10):1094-109. doi: 10.1097/BRS.0b013e3181a105fc.

25. Bokov A1, Isrelov A, Skorodumov A, Aleynik A, Simonov A, Mlyavykh S. An analysis of reasons for failed back surgery syndrome and partial results after different types of surgical lumbar nerve root decompression. Pain Physician. 2011 Nov-Dec;14(6):545-57.

26. Schwartzer et al. Prevalence and Clinical Features of Internal Disc Disruption in Patients with Chronic Low Back Pain. Spine 1995, vol 20 no 17, P1878-1883

Chapter 12

1. Kempke S1, Luyten P, Van Wambeke P, Coppens E, Morlion B. Self-critical perfectionism predicts outcome in multidisciplinary treatment for chronic pain. Pain

Pract. 2014 Apr;14(4):309-14. doi: 10.1111/papr.12071. Epub 2013 May 22.

2. Pinto A et al. Perfectionism in Chronic Pain: Are There Differences between fibromyalgia, Rheumatoid Arthritis and Healthy Controls? Ann Rheum Dis 2016;75:1190 doi:10.1136/annrheumdis-2016-eular.5668

3. Asghari, A., & Nicholas, M. K. (2006). Personality and pain-related beliefs/coping strategies: A prospective study. The Clinical Journal of Pain, 22, 10-18. doi:10.1097/01.ajp.0000146218.31780.0b

4. Hewitt, P. L., Flett, G. L., & Mikail, S. (1995). Perfectionism and relationship adjustment in pain patients and their spouses. Journal of Family Psychology, 9, 335-347. doi:10.1037/0893-3200.9.3.335

5. Hewitt, P. L, Flett, G. L., & Ediger, E. (1996). Perfectionism and depression: Longitudinal assessment of a specific vulnerability hypothesis. Journal of Abnormal Psychology, 105, 276-280. doi:10.1037/0021-843X.105.2.276

6. Elton, Deana, Gordon V. Stanley and Graham D. Burrows. 1978. Self Esteem and Chronic Pain. Journal of Psychosomatic Research 22: 25-31.

7. Hegarty D and Wall M. Prevalence of Stigmatization and Poor Self-esteem in Chronic Pain Patients. J Pain Relief 2014, 3:2 http://dx.doi.org/10.4172/2167-0846.1000136

8. Oswald, A. J. (2002), "Are you happy at work? Job satisfaction and work-life balance in the US and Europe", mimeo, University of Warwick.

9. Jonathan H. Westover. Potential Impacts of Globalization on Changing Job Quality and Worker

Satisfaction: A Descriptive Cross-National Comparative Examination.

10. John A. Bargh and Ezequiel Morsella. The Unconscious Mind. Perspect Psychol Sci. 2008 Jan; 3(1): 73–79. doi: 10.1111/j.1745-6916.2008.00064.x

11. Brill AA. Introduction. In: Brill AA, editor. The basic writings of Sigmund Freud. Modern Library; New York: 1938. pp. 1–32. Trans.

12. Schofferman, J., Anderson, D., Hines, R., Smith, G., & Keane, G. (1993). Childhood psychological trauma and chronic refractory low-back pain. The Clinical Journal of Pain, 9, 260-265

13. Domino, J. V., & Haber, J. D. (1987). Prior physical and sexual abuse in women with chronic headache: Clinical correlates. The Journal of Head and Face Pain, 27, 310-314.

14. Walling, M. K., Reiter, R. C., O'Hara, M. W., Milburn, A. K., Lilly, G., & Vincent, S. D. (1994). Abuse history and chronic pain in women: I. Prevalences of sexual abuse and physical abuse. Obstetrics & Gynecology, 84, 193-199.

15. Melzack, R., Coderre, T. J., Kat, J., & Vaccarino, A. L. (2001). Central neuroplasticity and pathological pain. Annals of the New York Academy of Sciences, 933, 157-174

16. Phillips, K. & Clauw, D. J. (2011). Central pain mechanisms in chronic pain states – maybe it is all in their head. Best Practice Research in Clinical Rheumatology, 25, 141-154.

17. Yunus, M. B. (2007). The role of central sensitization in symptoms beyond muscle pain, and the evaluation of a

patient with widespread pain. Best Practice Research in Clinical Rheumatology, 21, 481-497.

18. Apkarian V. Human Brain Imaging Studies of Chronic Pain.

19. L. Tiemann, E. S. May, M. Postorino, E. Schulz, M. M. Nickel, U. Bingel, M. Ploner, Differential neurophysiological correlates of bottom-up and top-down modulations of pain, Pain, 2015, Feb;156(2):289-96.

20. Apkarian AV. Pain perception in relation to emotional learning. Curr Opin Neurobiol. 2008;18:464–468.

21. Brickman P, Coates D, Janoff-Bulman R.Lottery winners and accident victims: is happiness relative? J Pers Soc Psychol. 1978 Aug;36(8):917-27.

Chapter 13

1. Massachusetts Institute of Technology. Two brain circuits involved with habitual learning. June 10, 2010

2. Ann M. Graybiel, The Basal Ganglia and Chunking of Action Repertoires, NEUROBIOLOGY OF LEARNING AND MEMORY 70, 119–136 (1998), ARTICLE NO. NL983843

3. Neville Owen, Geneviève N Healy, Charles E. Matthews, and David W. Dunstan. Too Much Sitting: The Population-Health Science of Sedentary Behavior. Exerc Sport Sci Rev. 2010 Jul; 38(3): 105–113. doi: 10.1097/JES.0b013e3181e373a2

4. Aviroop Biswas, BSc; Paul I. Oh, MD, MSc; Guy E. Faulkner, PhD; Ravi R. Bajaj, MD; Michael A. Silver, BSc; Marc S. Mitchell, MSc; David A. Alter, MD, PhD. Sedentary Time and Its Association With Risk for Disease Incidence, Mortality, and Hospitalization in

Adults: A Systematic Review and Meta-analysis. Annals of Internal Medicine. REVIEWS | 20 JANUARY 2015

5. Physical Activity 2016: Progress and Challenges. The Lancet. Published: July 27, 2016

6. Joan Vernikos, Ph.D. Sitting Kills, Moving Heals. December 2011

7. Rizolatti et al "The mirror neurone system" Annual review of Neuroscience 2004 27 [1] : 160-1932

8. Keysers et al "Mirror neurons" Current Biology 2010 19 [21]: R971-973

9. Crum AJ1, Langer EJ. Mind-set matters: exercise and the placebo effect. Psychol Sci. 2007 Feb;18(2):165-71.

Made in the USA
Coppell, TX
27 May 2021

56402359R00169